HEALTH AND THE ENVIRONMENT

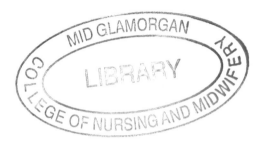

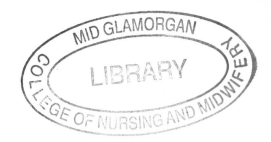
HEALTH AND THE ENVIRONMENT

FIONA GODLEE, MRCP

Assistant editor, British Medical Journal

and

ALISON WALKER, MRCP

Former editorial registrar, British Medical Journal

Now registrar in public health medicine,

Bloomsbury and Islington Health Authority

With an introduction by

SIR DONALD ACHESON, FRCP, FFPHM

Former Chief Medical Officer

Now visiting professor of international health,

London School of Hygiene and Tropical Medicine

Articles from the *British Medical Journal*

Published by the British Medical Journal
Tavistock Square, London WC1H 9JR

First published 1992

British Library Cataloguing-in-Publication Data.
A catalogue record for this book is available from the British Library.

ISBN 0–7279–0318–7

The following picture sources are acknowledged:

Page 1, Sheila Gray/Format; pages 4 and 50, Sally and Richard Greenhill; page 9, BMA News Review; page 12, Ron Gilling/Panos Pictures; page 19, Michael Harvey/Panos Pictures; page 22, Shahidul Alam/Panos Pictures; page 27, Maggie Murray/Format; page 30, National Aeronautics and Space Administration (NASA) GFSC/Science Photo Library; page 34, Sonia Miller/Environmental Picture Library; page 38, Barry Lewis/Network; page 44, Michael Abrahams/Network; page 53, Melanie Friend/Format; page 63, Michael Abrahams/Network; page 65, Tom Learmonth/Panos Pictures; page 68, Sally Bond/Environmental Picture Library; page 74, Honey Salvador/Network; page 87, National Rivers Authority; page 95, Paul Ferraby/Environmental Picture Library; page 104, Robert Brook/Environmental Picture Library; page 106, Patrick Piel/Gamma; and page 112, Hulton Picture Company.

Typeset by Bedford Typesetters Limited, Bedford
Printed and bound in Great Britain by
Latimer Trend & Company Ltd, Plymouth

Contents

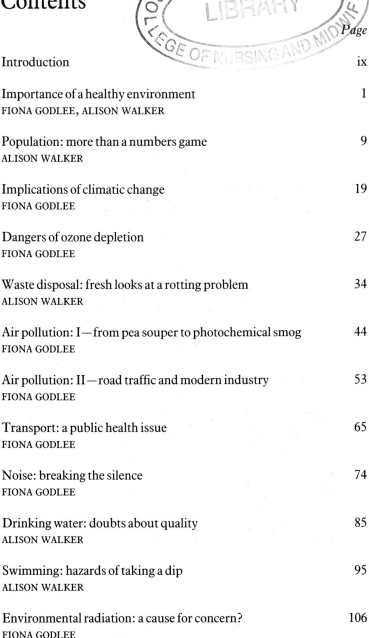

Page

Introduction ix

Importance of a healthy environment 1
FIONA GODLEE, ALISON WALKER

Population: more than a numbers game 9
ALISON WALKER

Implications of climatic change 19
FIONA GODLEE

Dangers of ozone depletion 27
FIONA GODLEE

Waste disposal: fresh looks at a rotting problem 34
ALISON WALKER

Air pollution: I — from pea souper to photochemical smog 44
FIONA GODLEE

Air pollution: II — road traffic and modern industry 53
FIONA GODLEE

Transport: a public health issue 65
FIONA GODLEE

Noise: breaking the silence 74
FIONA GODLEE

Drinking water: doubts about quality 85
ALISON WALKER

Swimming: hazards of taking a dip 95
ALISON WALKER

Environmental radiation: a cause for concern? 106
FIONA GODLEE

Introduction

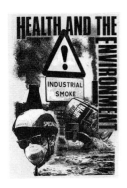

As the first country to industrialise, Britain was soon confronted within its rapidly growing cities by the grim effects of the deteriorating environment on health. As early as 1842 Edwin Chadwick in his report, *The Sanitary Condition of the Labouring Population*, drew attention to the relation between overcrowding, accumulation of excrement, and lack of clean water and the incidence of disease and premature death. His survey had a profound impact and led on to the sanitary revolution. When the first comprehensive analyses of mortality within the cities became available these confirmed "the inequality with which deaths are distributed in different districts," and in 1858 in his first report John Simon drew the firm conclusion that the observed excesses were largely due to environmental and social deficiencies "which could be remedied" (such as ill ventilated and crowded buildings and neglect of children).

But in the 1850s the world contained only about a billion people. At this level of population the oceans and the air were still sufficient to dilute and absorb waste and the consumption of the world's renewable resources was not beyond its capacity for regeneration. In recent years concern about the consequences for the global ecosystem of the consumption of energy by the world's escalating population—currently just short of 5·5 billion and likely to reach 10 billion by the year 2050—and the accumulation of its waste has forced the United Nations urgently to reappraise the effect of the environment on health.

In 1987 the Brundtland Commission's report, *Our Common Future*, urged that the present generation should so order and contain its economic development as to bequeath the environment in a healthy condition to its successors. This theme is taken up again and applied specifically to health in *Implementation of the Global Strategy for Health for All by the Year 2000*, a remarkable report just published by the World Health Organisation's Commission on Health and Environment as its main contribution to the United Nations conference on environment and development (Rio de Janeiro, June 1992). The report concludes that although there is a powerful synergy between health, environmental protection, and sustainable use of resources, health has rarely received due consideration or priority in environmental or development programmes.

The report points to three main global objectives. The first is to achieve a sustainable basis for health for all by slowing down and then halting population growth as soon as possible and by promoting patterns of consumption among the affluent which are consistent with ecological sustainability. The second is to provide an environment which promotes health, and the third to make all individuals and organisations aware of their responsibility for health and for its environmental basis.

In the pursuit of the third objective—a wider awareness—the *British Medical Journal*'s series of articles, *Health and the Environment*, is particularly timely. In the space of 12 articles the authors cover a great deal of ground. The first three describe vividly how man, the main cause of environmental degradation, "has become its principal victim." Thus while the estimates of the growth of the world's population are revised upwards and the profligate consumption of energy continues to escalate, the spread of deserts due to altered rainfall patterns, land degradation, ozone depletion, and acid rain are already threatening food production. Already a fifth of the world's population lacks sufficient food. As far as water is concerned, the International Drinking Water Supply and Sanitation Decade, which ended in 1990, extended safe water supplies to 81% of urban dwellers and 58% of rural inhabitants, but because of further population increase the absolute number of people still without access to this basic service has continued to grow.

On global warming the authors conclude that although the case for an upward trend is not yet proved beyond doubt, the potential risks to health, indeed to survival itself, for many millions of people are so dire that "as with acute medical emergencies there is no time to wait for the return of the investigations which would confirm the diagnosis." Unfortunately there is little evidence that national governments have so far given much heed to this message. The United States Environmental Protection Agency has estimated that to stabilise atmospheric carbon dioxide emissions will have to be cut by at least a half, but Britain has agreed only to stabilise emissions by 2005 and the United States has so far refused to agree any limits at all.

One of the more controversial themes of the articles is the attribution to the car and private motoring of an almost criminal role in the deterioration of environmental health. The world's 400 million car fleet not only provides the largest single component of photochemical smog and consumes far more energy/passenger/km travelled than most forms of public transport, but at the same time is creating escalating problems of traffic congestion and noise in cities. Motor cars also consume a phenomenal amount of space, and within Los Angeles, for example, no less than two thirds of that huge city's land area is given up to motorways, other roads, and parking lots. In many parts of the world the car also dictates overall urban planning and transport policies are in favour of the car owner. Thus in terms of recreation facilities and shops offering cheap and healthy foods the choice offered to the car owner is usually much greater than to households without cars (in Britain two fifths of the total).

The book also deals with several other environmental issues, such as the dangers of ozone depletion, waste disposal (including the problems of clinical waste), and noise. Its crucial paradigm is the currently unstable relation between population, health, and a sustainable environment. One implication of the instability is that there is an urgent need for a new approach to equity between the developed and developing world so that wealth currently lost in waste and overconsumption can in future be invested to reduce poverty and ignorance. Furthermore, from now on new development policies must be assessed for their impact on health as well as on the environment. The achievement of these aims will require major changes in the attitudes of individuals as well as of governments. At the political level within the European Community the draft Treaty of European Union (Maastricht treaty) provides a glimmer of hope. For, in addition to bringing health protection within the competence of the community, article 129 provides that the requirement to protect health shall form a constituent of the community's other policies. But it remains to be seen to what extent the new health council will make an effective input to the work of other councils such as those concerned with industry and agriculture in this context. Health professionals as advocates and agents for both private and public health have a key part to play in drawing attention to the serious and growing threat to global health occasioned by our "energy hungry and throwaway society."

SIR DONALD ACHESON

Acknowledgments

We thank Mr Timothy Dyson of the London School of Economics and Political Sciences for his help in compiling the chapter on population; Professor Andrew Haines and Dr Jonathan Cowie for their help with the chapter on the health implications of climatic change; Dr Robin Russell Jones for his help with the chapter on ozone depletion; Tara Lamont of the BMA and William Townend of the London Waste Regulation Authority for their help with the chapter on waste disposal; and Dr Malcolm Green, Fiona Wier of Friends of the Earth, Dr Lutz Blank of Environmental Resources Limited, Dr Simon Wolff, Dr Peter Burney, and Dr Andrew Wardlaw for their help with the chapters on air pollution. For the chapter on transport we drew heavily on the work of the Transport and Health Study Group in Britain and of Marcia Lowe in the United States; we also thank Dr Simon Wolff. The London Cycling Campaign can be contacted on 071 928 7220. We thank Dr Adrian Davis and Professor Chris Rice for their help in preparing the chapter on noise, Professor Ronald Packham for his help with the chapter on drinking water, Dr Edmund Pike for his help with the chapter on swimming, and the National Radiological Protection Board and Hazel Inskip for their help with the chapter on radiation.

Importance of a healthy environment

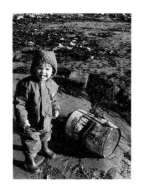

FIONA GODLEE,
ALISON WALKER

Doctors seem to spend their time these days exhorting their patients to adopt healthier habits: to exercise more, eat less, drink only a little, and smoke not at all; to wear seat belts, crash helmets, and condoms. But perhaps the most important risks to health are beyond people's immediate control, caused by the unhealthy habits not of individuals but of an energy hungry and throwaway society.

The environmental price

Since the industrial revolution and the advent of the internal combustion engine we have consumed the earth's natural resources and altered our environment at a rate never seen before. The demand for energy is constantly growing, fuelled by the world's escalating population—now at 5·3 billion and estimated to reach 10 billion by 2050.[1] In 1989 the world's energy consumption reached 9300 million tons of oil equivalent, causing the emission of nearly six billion tons of carbon into the environment (figure).[2] The World Energy Conference concluded that by 2020 the world would be using 75% more energy, and most of it would still be supplied by coal, oil, and nuclear power.[3]

The destructive consequences of human industry on the environment are in many cases already evident, in others controversial. Chlorofluorocarbons, still used as a propellant in aerosols in some countries and in the manufacture of refrigerators, are destroying the

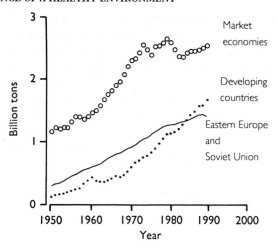

Carbon emissions from fossil fuels 1950-1989. From "State of the World 1991"[2]

layer of ozone in the outer atmosphere which protects the earth from the sun's ultraviolet rays. If levels of chlorofluorocarbons continue to rise at the present rate—about 3% a year—a 6% reduction in stratospheric ozone has been predicted by 2040.[4] The resultant increase in the amount of ultraviolet B reaching the earth's surface—1·5-2% for every 1% reduction in total column ozone—has the potential to cause ecological catastrophe. Phytoplankton, for example, the basis of the food chain for all aquatic creatures, are highly vulnerable to damage from ultraviolet B radiation.[5]

Greenhouse gases—carbon dioxide from the burning of fossil fuels, methane, nitrous oxide, and chlorofluorocarbons—are accumulating in the outer atmosphere, where concentrations of carbon dioxide are now higher than at any time in the past 160 000 years.[6] There is now overwhelming scientific consensus that this is causing global warming.[6a] The earth's surface temperature has risen by about 0·6°C in the past 100 years and further increases of 2-5°C have been predicted over the next 50 to 100 years, causing potentially catastrophic rises in sea level.[5]

Road vehicles, responsible for emitting a fifth of the anthropogenic carbon dioxide in air, also produce acidic gases—nitrogen oxides and sulphur dioxide—which cause acid rain. Though heavy industry is bringing its emissions under control, the use of road transport is increasing at a rate likely to swamp any reductions in pollution achieved by technological improvements in car engines. The Department of Transport estimates that in Britain the number of vehicle miles will double by 2025, causing an estimated doubling of emissions of carbon dioxide.[7] For the same reason emissions of nitrogen oxides, which are predicted to fall over the next 20 years owing to the introduction of catalytic converters, will be on the increase again by 2020.

Acid rain lays waste large areas of agricultural land and forest, adding to deforestation caused by harvesting hardwood and the pressure for more agricultural land. Each year an area of tropical forest the size of Austria is destroyed.[1] Deforestation increases the build up of carbon dioxide because trees fix carbon from the air. It also spells disaster for biological diversity as more than half the species on earth live in the tropical rain forests.[8]

The human price

Man, the main cause of environmental degradation, is also one of its victims. Apart from the direct effects that increases in ambient temperature might have on health — higher mortality from heart and lung disease; the spread of tropical diseases to temperate climates; and more deaths, disability, and psychological problems due to storms and natural disasters — global warming would cause the sea to expand and swamp large areas of habitable and agricultural land.[9] A rise in sea level of one metre (the International Panel on Climate Change's 1990 estimate[10]) would affect five million square kilometres of the world's lowest lying land, causing the loss of one third of our crop growing areas and creating 50 million environmental refugees.[6]

Nuclear energy reduces reliance on fossil fuels but creates problems of its own. The fire at Chernobyl nuclear power station in 1986 is still having repercussions in parts of Europe, and smaller leaks of radiation are a cause of anxiety after reports of clusters of leukaemia in children living near nuclear installations in Britain.[11-13]

Thinning of the ozone layer will increase the incidence of sun related skin cancers. A 10% reduction in total column ozone — possible by the late twenty first century if levels of chlorofluorocarbons continue to increase at their present rate — could result in an extra 160 000 cases of non-melanocytic skin cancer in the United States each year and an extra 4000 deaths from malignant melanoma.[14] At the moment the incidence of melanoma in the United States is a quarter the incidence in Queensland, Australia, where about one in every 150 white males dies of the disease.

3

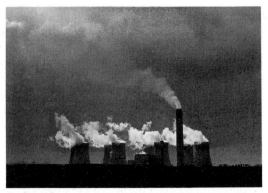

Perhaps the most important risks to health are caused by an energy hungry society

Man's love affair with the motor car is also turning sour. City smogs, once thought to be a thing of the past, are back again. The impenetrable pea soupers, such as the one which enveloped London in December 1952, killing 4000 people,[15] were caused by domestic and industrial burning of high sulphur coal. In their place there is now an invisible cocktail of pollutants emitted from road vehicles, many of which are known to be harmful to health.[16] Nitrogen dioxide and sulphur dioxide are respiratory irritants. They are the main constituents of acid rain and exacerbate asthma and chronic lung disease. Airborne particulates, emitted mainly from diesel vehicles and visible in the air as black smoke, are inhaled into the lungs and carry with them acidic gases and volatile organic compounds such as benzene, which is a known carcinogen. Ozone at ground level, produced by the effects of sunlight on traffic fumes, causes impaired lung function, and there is some evidence that the increase in air pollution over the past 40 years could be responsible for an increase in the number of admissions to hospital and deaths caused by asthma.[17]

The waste products of industrial processes, domestic consumption, and transport are creating further health risks. In England and Wales alone some 2·5 billion tonnes of waste are disposed of every year, about 90% of which ends up in one of the 4000 controlled landfill sites around the country.[18] There have not been many studies on the health risks associated with waste disposal, but there is some evidence that refuse workers are at increased risk of illness.[19]

Air pollution, ozone depletion, land degradation, acid rain, and altered rainfall patterns have caused a reduction in world harvests

4

and fears of a world food crisis. The world's grain harvest currently increases by an average of 15 million tons each year.[9] This is already well below the 28 million ton increase needed to keep pace with population growth. But if current rates of environmental degradation continue, the world's grain harvest could fall by about 14 million tons each year. Famine stricken countries that rely on food imports from the West are the most at risk—and the least able to manage.

Reversing the damage

Reversing damage to the environment will take time. It is not just a question of removing the remaining sources of pollution but of dealing with the stockpile of pollutants that have accumulated over the years. Toxins in landfill sites, for example, continue to leach slowly into ground water, and non-biodegradable pesticides are still working their way down the food chain.

It may not be possible to reverse the damage in our lifetime or even that of our children and grandchildren. Carbon dioxide and chlorofluorocarbons, both of which have long half lives, persist in the atmosphere long after they are produced. Half of the carbon dioxide emitted since the start of the industrial revolution remains in the atmosphere today.[6] Chlorofluorocarbons linger for 50 to 100 years before they are broken down, and even with reductions in emissions in line with the Montreal protocol, active chlorine levels in the stratosphere will roughly double by 2040.[20] Alternatives to both chlorofluorocarbons and the burning of fossil fuels already exist, but adopting them on a worldwide scale requires planning and financial investment. Countries in the Third World are recent converts to cars, tin cans, and aerosol sprays. Increasingly in debt to the West, they cannot afford to modernise their now outdated technology. They will need help to make the switch to more environmentally friendly methods.

As the paths of the rich and poor nations continue to diverge the task of controlling the world's population will become more, not less, difficult. The population of western Europe is falling. By the end of the century only 20% of the world's population will be living in developed countries.[21] But the ability to limit family size stems partly from the knowledge that children will survive to adulthood. In developing countries family planning must be accompanied by efforts to reduce child mortality and improve the health of women.

For many people in the West environmental priorities are quite different. They have shifted from global issues to the luxury of questioning the quality of tap water or the level of air pollution in cities. While scientists continue to argue that tap water in Britain is just as safe today as it was 50 years ago, the public expresses its doubts by buying bottled water at 1000 times the price. Sales of bottled mineral water increased from three million to 128 million litres between 1976 and 1986.[22]

Epidemiological evidence to confirm or refute the public's fears about the safety of tap water is largely lacking, but some aspects of environmental research are coming up with answers. Swimming in sea water contaminated by raw sewage has been shown, through a number of studies since the 1970s, to be associated with increased risk of gastrointestinal symptoms and ear, nose, and throat infections.[23] As a result efforts are now being made to clean up beaches in Britain and Europe, prompted by European Community directives and the fear of losing income from tourists.

Quality of the evidence

It would be nice to be able to say with certainty that x amount of air pollutant causes y additional cases of asthma each year. Unfortunately, when it comes to environmental pollution it is not quite so simple. Predictions about global warming and ozone depletion are based on mathematical models, which are open to question. Equally uncertain are estimates of the effects on health of chemical pollutants, airborne carcinogens, and radiation in the environment. These are largely based on the evidence of occupational studies and "natural" disasters such as the explosion of the atomic bomb in Hiroshima and the accidental contamination of the water supply with aluminium sulphate at the Lowermoor works in Camelford in 1988. But there are problems in extrapolating from short term, high dose exposure to long term, low dose, environmental exposure. Large scale population studies that should circumvent these problems are often flawed by, for example, the difficulty of finding control subjects who have not also been exposed to the environmental pollutant.

In the next few chapters we examine the risks to human health from environmental pollution. Starting with the population growth which primes the pump, we then consider the possible impact of climatic change due to global warming and the destruction of the ozone layer. Subsequent chapters deal with the related issues of air pollution, transport, and environmental noise and with the quality of drinking water, the standard of beaches, and the disposal of sewage and hazardous waste. Finally we ask whether radiation in the environment, whether natural or man made, is dangerous to health.

These questions are of great importance to doctors. Understanding the effects of the environment on health allows the practice of perhaps the ultimate in preventive medicine. We may already be treating health problems related to environmental pollution: asthma and bronchitis from city smogs, gastrointestinal and ear infections from polluted sea water, hearing loss and psychological problems caused by environmental noise. Some questions remain unanswered. Does air pollution cause lung cancer? Is the nuclear industry the cause of leukaemia clusters in children? What are the risks from contaminated drinking water and radon in homes? Patients are increasingly well informed on these issues, but they expect doctors to provide information and advice. Doctors are in a prime position not only to monitor the effects of environmental pollution on their patients but to change the behaviour of individuals and those in authority. It is only through radical change that environmental degradation and its damaging effects on human health will be halted.

1 United Nations Population Fund. *The state of world population 1991*. New York: United Nations Population Fund, 1991.

2 Brown LR. The new world order. In: Brown LR, ed. *State of the world 1991. A Worldwatch Institute report on progress toward a sustainable society*. London: Earthscan Publications, 1991.

3 Flavin C, Lenssen N. Designing a sustainable energy system. In: Brown LR, ed. *State of the world 1991. A Worldwatch Institute report on progress toward a sustainable society*. London: Earthscan Publications, 1991.

4 Watson RT. Present state of knowledge of the ozone layer. In: Russell Jones R, Wigley T, eds. *Ozone depletion: health and environmental consequences*. Chichester: Wiley, 1989.

5 Leaf A. Potential health effects of global climatic and environmental changes. *N Engl J Med* 1989;**321**:1577-83.

6 Brown LR, ed. *State of the world 1989: a Worldwatch Institute report on progress toward a sustainable society*. New York: W W Norton, 1989.

6a Intergovernmental Panel on Climate Change. *Climate change*. Cambridge: Cambridge University Press, 1990.

7 Fergusson M, Holman C, Barrett M. *Atmospheric emissions from the use of transport in the UK*. Vol 1. *The estimation of current and future emissions*. London: World Wildlife Fund and Earth Resources Research, 1989.

8 Wilson EO. Threats to biodiversity. *Sci Am* 1989;**261**:108-16.

9 Haines A. Potential impacts on health of atmospheric change. *J Public Health Med* 1991;**13**:69-80.

10 Houghton JT, Jenkins GJ, Ephraums JJ. *Climate change—the IPCC scientific assessment*. Cambridge: Cambridge University Press, 1990.

11 Independent Advisory Group. *Investigation of the possible increased incidence of cancer in West Cumbria*. London: HMSO, 1984. (Black report.)

12 Committee on Medical Aspects of Radiation in the Environment. *Investigation of the possible increased incidence of leukaemia in young people near the Dounreay Nuclear Establishment, Caithness, Scotland.* London: HMSO, 1988.

13 Committee on Medical Aspects of Radiation in the Environment. *Report on the incidence of childhood cancer in the west Berkshire and north Hampshire area, in which are situated the Atomic Weapons Research Establishment, Aldermaston, and the Royal Ordnance Factory, Burghfield.* London: HMSO, 1989.

14 Russell Jones R. Consequences for human health of stratospheric ozone depletion. In: Russell Jones R, Wigley T, eds. *Ozone depletion: health and environmental consequences.* Chichester: Wiley, 1989.

15 Ministry of Health. *Mortality and morbidity during the London fog of December 1952.* London: HMSO, 1954.

16 World Health Organisation. *Air quality guidelines for Europe.* Copenhagen: WHO Regional Publications, 1987.

17 Read C. *Air pollution and health.* London: Greenpeace, 1991.

18 British Medical Association. *Hazardous waste and human health.* Oxford: Oxford University Press, 1991.

19 Gustavsson P. Mortality among workers at a municipal waste incinerator. *Am J Ind Med* 1989;**15**:245-53.

20 Elman RS, Pyle JA. Numerical modelling of ozone perturbations. In: Russell Jones R, Wigley T, eds. *Ozone depletion: health and environmental consequences.* Chichester: Wiley, 1989.

21 United Nations Department of International Economic and Social Affairs. *World population at the turn of the century.* New York: United Nations, 1989.

22 Wheeler D. *Risk assessment and the public perception of water quality. Annual symposium of the Institution of Water and Environmental Management.* London, 1990:2-1–2-13.

23 Pike EB. *Health effects of sea bathing. Phase 1—pilot study at Langland Bay.* Medmenham: Water Research Centre, 1990. (Report DoE 2518 M(P).)

Population: more than a numbers game

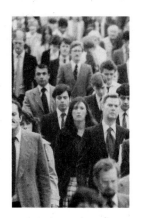

ALISON WALKER

On 11 July 1987 the world's population officially reached five billion—a landmark date. But the peak has not yet been reached. Numbers are still rising and estimates have again been revised upwards. The latest projections from the United Nations Population Fund now put the world's population at 10 billion by 2050.[1]

But the earth cannot sustain an ever increasing rise in world population. Already the effect is taking its toll on the environment; global warming, ozone depletion, and acid rain have all been caused by man through industrial expansion; and overexploitation of land in the Third World has caused grasslands to deteriorate, soil erosion to increase, and land to be slowly converted to desert. In terms of human need, the long term effects of environmental change are still being debated, but a more urgent concern is now being raised. Environmental changes are already affecting agriculture and are threatening food production all over the world. Harvests are suffering, and estimates show that the current food production is leaving one fifth of the world's current population without enough food.[2]

The cause is not simply maldistribution. After a record grain harvest in 1986, absolute grain production worldwide dropped by 5% in 1987 and by a further 5% in 1988, when the grain harvests of the United States, Canada, the Soviet Union, and China suffered from severe drought and crop failure. Meanwhile the world's population grew by 3·6% in 1987 and 1988. The United States' grain harvest was

TABLE 1 – *Crude estimate of additional loss of world grain output each year as result of environmental degradation*[3]

Form of degradation	Grain output loss (million tons)
Land degradation:	
Soil erosion	9
Waterlogging and salting of irrigated land	1
Loss of soil organic matter from burning cow dung and crop residue	
Shortening of shifting cultivation cycle	2*
Compaction of soil from heavy equipment	
Crop damage:	
Air pollution	1
Flooding	
Acid rain	1*
Increased ultraviolet radiation	
Total	14

*Because lack of data makes it difficult to quantify the crop losses from these three sources their effect is estimated collectively.

affected the most, falling by 27% in 1988 compared with the previous year. Over 100 nations depend on food imports from the United States, and only the large reserves have prevented a serious food crisis. Africa is more dependent than most, not only having the highest population growth anywhere in the world but also declining food production. Civil wars in Ethiopia, the Sudan, and elsewhere over the past two decades have resulted in widespread famines as local crops have been damaged and transport routes for food donations disrupted.

Falling food production

Despite estimates indicating a return of food production to 1986 levels there is still a need to replenish lost food reserves. A review of the world's food supply suggests that the world could be losing 14 million additional tons of grain output each year because of environmental damage to land and crops (table I).[3]

Soil erosion, for example, is estimated to be reducing the productivity of one third of the world's cropland. In India an estimated six billion tons of topsoil—the equivalent of 21 000 km² of arable land—is

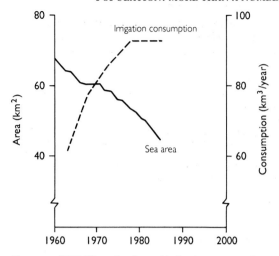

Sea area, 1960-85, and estimated irrigation consumption, 1963-87, in Aral Sea basin[3]

being lost every year. Land irrigation without adequate drainage is also affecting food production, causing waterlogging and salting as water evaporates and concentrates salts in the upper few layers of soil. Vast areas of the United States and Soviet Union have been made unproductive in this way. The Aral Sea region of the Soviet Union, for example, has been turned into an ecological disaster by the diversion of rivers to irrigate the surrounding farmland (fig). The sea is drying up, and the irrigated cropland has been turned into a salt desert. Dust, dried pesticides, and salt have been carried thousands of miles away by winds and rain.

Each year some 3300 km^3 of water are removed from the earth's rivers, streams, and underground aquifers to water crops. Water is being drawn from aquifers faster than it is being replaced, and in the United States more than four million hectares are watered by pumping in excess of replenishment. Deforestation is also taking its toll, increasing the run off of water from land and altering the pattern of recycling of rainfall on to cropland. Air pollution from cars and coal fired power stations is also damaging crops, ozone causing by far the most harm. And sensitive crops such as soya beans are being destroyed by the rise in ultraviolet radiation caused by depletion of the ozone layer in the upper stratosphere.[23]

The green revolution has been responsible for the bigger world

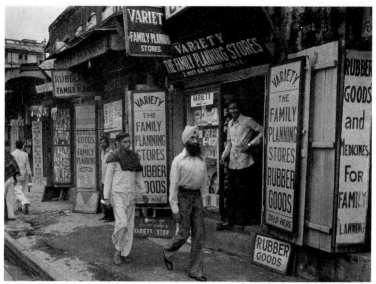

Demand for contraception around the world has never been higher

harvests of the past four or five decades as the result of advances in science and agriculture. But it cannot be guaranteed to continue. Farmers in the Third World may still be helped to improve food production, not only through biotechnology but by protecting soil and restoring the productivity of degraded land. But if the gap between food production and demand is to be narrowed, then the population question also needs to be tackled.

Population side of the food equation

Current indicators show a continuing fall in the rate of growth of the world's population, both in developed countries and in the Third World.[4] This has been caused by a worldwide fall in birth rate first noticed between 1960 and 1970. The world growth rate reached an all time high in the late 1960s at 2·04%. Since then it has fallen, and in the mid-1980s was only 1·67%

A falling growth rate does not, however, mean that the world's population problems are over. Far from it. Population growth is exponential and will continue to rise even if birth rates fall, although at a slower rate. Projections from the United Nations suggest that population growth may continue until the twenty second century and may not level off until it reaches 11·6 billion.[1]

The growth rates in industrialised and Third World countries are diverging (table II). By 2025 the population of the industrialised countries will have fallen from a third to less than a fifth of the world's population while the Third World will have increased its share of the population to more than 80%. A greater fall in birth rates in developed countries partly accounts for this change. Low birth rates are responsible for the growth rates of only 1% a year or less now found in the United States, Australia, and New Zealand.[1] In Europe the birth rate has declined from 2·1 births per woman in 1965 (the rate needed to maintain the size of its population) to only 1·7, causing Europe to slip from 15·6% of the world population in 1950 to 10·2% in 1985. Migration into Europe means that the population will not fall, but migrants from poor to rich countries pose an additional environmental threat, taking on the lifestyle of their adopted country, consuming resources, and causing environmental damage. But there is a positive side to this migration as the departure of people from the Third World reduces demand in their countries of origin.

The picture is quite different for the developing countries, where the total birth rate, although falling, was still over four births per woman in the early 1980s. At least 95% of the projected increase in growth of the world's population will take place in developing countries, which are growing at a rate of at least 2·5% a year, this adding some 65 million people a year to their populations.[5]

TABLE 2—*Evolution of the world's population, by main region.*[4] *Figures are numbers in millions (percentages)*

	1950	1985	2000	2025
World	2 516	4 837	6 122	8 206
Developed countries	832 (33·1)	1 174 (24·3)	1 277 (20·9)	1 396 (17·0)
Developing countries	1 684 (66·9)	3 663 (75·7)	4 846 (79·2)	6 809 (83·0)
Africa	224 (8·9)	555 (11·5)	872 (14·2)	1 617 (19·7)
Latin America	165 (6·6)	405 (8·4)	546 (8·9)	779 (9·5)
Asia	1 376 (54·7)	2 818 (58·3)	3 549 (58·0)	4 535 (55·3)
China	555 (22·1)	1 060 (21·9)	1 256 (20·5)	1 475 (18·0)
India	358 (14·2)	759 (15·7)	964 (15·8)	1 229 (15·0)
Europe	392 (15·6)	492 (10·2)	512 (8·4)	524 (6·4)
United States	152 (6·0)	238 (4·9)	268 (4·4)	312 (3·8)
Soviet Union	180 (7·2)	278 (5·7)	315 (5·1)	368 (4·5)

Africa is experiencing the largest growth rate ever seen anywhere in the world. By the end of the century its population will have reached 900 million—250 million more than today—representing a growth rate of 3% per year. Asia still has more than half of the world's population, although its growth rate is much less than that of Africa. Population growth on this scale has forced previously self sufficient rural populations to overexploit their farm lands. An estimated 580 million people are living in absolute poverty on marginal or fragile land. One of the results has been mass migration from subsistence farming to the cities.

Explosive urban growth is now being seen in almost all parts of the developing world, particularly in places like Mexico City, Cairo, and São Paolo. More than 85 countries have city populations double those of 10 years ago, and by the end of the century the urban population of the developing world will be almost double that of the developed world.[1] Inadequate sanitation, housing, food, and water all contribute to a desperate situation in which social and political troubles frequently ensue. But why has the birth rate of the developed world fallen so much more than that of the Third World? Answering this question will provide some clues as to ways of controlling population growth.

Controlling population growth

Controlling the population growth in the Third World is, unfortunately, not that easy. While the developed world has managed to reduce both its birth and its death rates, the Third World is still experiencing falling death rates coupled with high (and in some places rising) birth rates (box). Social and political instability, falling per person incomes, declining agricultural productivity, and landlessness in the Third World all need to be tackled if its soaring population is to be reduced.

Not least of the hurdles to be overcome in the developing world is inadequate health care. Already hampered by widespread malnutrition, contaminated water supplies, and poor sanitaton, it is now further burdened by the speed with which the AIDS epidemic is taking hold, particularly in Africa. Projections from the United Nations predict that even in the worst scenario—if HIV seroprevalence reached 21% by the year 2000, implying an AIDS related death rate of 12 per 1000 population—the population of Africa will still be increasing at the turn of the century.[1] But even they recognise

The demographic trap

In 1945 Notestein described a theoretical model of demographic transition to a stable equilibrium of low birth and death rates. The model gave three stages.

• Birth rates and death rates are high and the population grows slowly if at all

• Living and health conditions improve and death rates fall, but birth rates remain high and the population grows rapidly

• Economic and social gains combine to reduce birth rates, and, as in the first stage, birth rates and death rates are in equilibrium, but at a much lower level.

This picture was based on the experience in Europe, where transition to the third stage happened in the nineteenth century. Many Third World countries today, however, have fallen into a demographic trap unforeseen by Notestein, failing to complete the transition and reach the third stage.[6] Unable to achieve the social and economic gains necessary to reduce births, they ultimately experience a rise in their death rates again. The population reaches an unsustainable state, with a high birth rate and death rate and increasing pressure on its resources. Although there is little evidence for this "trap," the possibility of such processes is worth considering.

that this estimate does not take into account the crippling effect that the epidemic will have on the already suffering health care system.

Aid programmes

Relief agencies, attempting to battle with the problems of the Third World, have come to recognise the need to integrate aid programmes. Population control through family planning, in particular, will not succeed unless other issues are also addressed. Unicef strongly emphasises the importance of combining family planning with primary health care.[7] It sees family planning as one of four synergistic measures—the others being economic progress, improvements for women, and reduced child mortality—which act to reduce birth rates.

Infant mortality is particularly contentious. Maurice King, consultant public health physician in Leeds, questions the point of improving the health of infants in Third World countries when it is not matched by other efforts.[8] "Such measures as oral rehydration should not be introduced on a public health scale," he writes, "since they increase the man-years of human misery, ultimately from starvation." Unicef, however, stresses the importance of reducing child death rates in order to achieve lower birth rates. Firstly, it says, an infant death ends the suppression of ovulation which is caused by breast feeding. Secondly, the death of a child can prompt couples to replace the loss by a new pregnancy, and, thirdly, when child death rates are high many parents anticipate loss of their children by having more than they actually want.

Family planning

Some countries have reduced birth rates by successfully integrating family planning into the primary health care system. In Sri Lanka, for example, emphasis has been placed on women's development and maternal and child health alongside family planning. Female literacy rates are in excess of 80% and contraceptives are now used regularly by almost 70% of the population.[1]

Effective family planning is still used by only just over half of all married couples in developing countries.[1] Clearly use needs to increase, but getting the message across is difficult. Cultural beliefs that sterility is a curse need to be discussed with care, but other social, religious, and political barriers also need to be surmounted.

China managed to reduce its birth rate much faster than anyone would have thought possible. The successful reduction of the birth rate from 4·74 at the beginning of the 1970s to 2·36 just 10 years later had much to do with family planning being a "civic duty" under the Chinese constitution.[4] Families who complied were rewarded with incentives—including better housing, better educational facilities, free child care, paid time off for abortions and sterilisations, and paid maternity leave.[2] Although the programme was extremely successful, by the end of the 1970s the population had climbed to one billion. In 1979 the one child family was made the official "goal" for 50% of all couples and two children for the rest. With these additional measures the average family size had fallen to just 2·1 by the mid-1980s. But family planning in most developing countries does not have the political support given to it in China, and there are humanitarian problems with this approach.[8a]

The exclusive support of family planning as part of primary health services can be hampered by ill equipped clinics staffed by underpaid government workers.[9] Other channels for distributing contraceptives do exist and in many cases community based schemes through non-government organisations are more effective. In Nigeria, for example, the familiarity and accessibility of the markets make them a more successful means of distributing contraceptives—even though they are not free—than the local family planning association.[1]

Any investment in family planning is increasingly likely to succeed —figures show that demands for contraceptives around the world have never been so high. According to a survey carried out by the United Nations, a large proportion of married women in the Third World do not want any more children—the figures ranging from 12% in the Ivory Coast to 77% in the Republic of Korea.[4]

Support from industrialised countries

The United Nations Population Fund has set targets for slowing the growth of the world's population. Its long term aim is to ensure that family planning services are available to all couples, but it has set a short term target of making them available to 567 million couples —59% of all married women of reproductive age—by the year 2000. This will help ensure a fall in total birth rate in developing countries from 3·8 to 3·3 children per woman.[1]

To meet its target the population fund will require a doubling of its funding to $9bn annually by the year 2000, half of which will have to come from the international community. Current support given by industrialised nations varies, but it is still pitifully low.[10] In 1990 only 0·9% of the total development assistance budget provided by industrialised nations was spent on population or family programmes.

Financial aid is not the only way the developed world can help the Third World. One of the greatest contributions it can make is to ensure that the Third World learns from the industrialised world's mistakes. There seems little point in industrialised countries trying to extricate themselves from the effects of the damage they have caused to the environment if the mistakes are simply going to be repeated by the Third World.

Two hundred years after Thomas Malthus, population growth remain's a problem. Three interlinked issues—food, health, and family planning—are all central to the population issue, and the lack of them is felt most acutely in the Third World. Population control is an urgent problem which should not be neglected, nor confined to Third World debates. Everyone—especially doctors as part of their public health duty—should make population growth as much a public concern as global warming, acid rain, and other ecological issues.[11]

At the end of the day, however, it will be the political and economic motives of politicians which decide the fate of the world's population.

1 United Nations Population Fund. *The state of world population 1991*. New York: United Nations Population Fund, 1991.
2 Ehrlich PR, Ehrlich AH. *The population explosion*. New York: Simon and Schuster, 1990.
3 Worldwatch Institute. *State of the world 1990*. New York: N W Norton, 1990.
4 United Nations Department of International Economic and Social Affairs. *World population at the turn of the century*. New York: United Nations, 1989.
5 World Health Organisation. *From Alma ata to the year 2000: reflections at the midpoint*. Geneva: WHO, 1988.
6 Brown L. Analysing the demographic trap. In: *The state of the world 1987*. New York: N W Norton, 1987.
7 Unicef. *The state of the world's children 1991*. Oxford: Oxford University Press, 1991.
8 King M. Health is a sustainable state. *Lancet* 1990;**336**:664-7.
8a Jarmulowicz M. Health and the environment: population. *BMJ* 1991;**303**:1547.
9 Nothing is unthinkable. *Lancet* 1990;**336**:659-61.
10 Potts M, Rosenfield A. The fifth freedom revisited. 1. Background and existing programmes. *Lancet* 1990;**336**:1227-31.
11 Smith T. The population bomb has exploded already. *BMJ* 1990;**301**:681-2.

Implications of climatic change

FIONA GODLEE

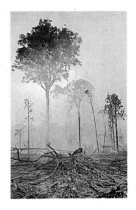

Every age has its catastrophe theory. In the past decade alone scientists have threatened us with a new ice age and a nuclear winter. Now two new threats confront us, global warming and the destruction of the ozone layer, linked by their origin in man's pollution of the environment. Both have enormous implications for health. This chapter examines the potential impacts of global warming on health. The next chapter examines the dangers of ozone depletion.

Global warming

Without some form of insulating layer to trap heat from the sun the earth could not sustain life. Its surface temperature would be 40°C lower and the oceans would freeze.[1] Insulation, largely in the form of atmospheric carbon dioxide, allows the passage of visible and ultra-violet light from the sun while preventing too much of the solar heat that radiates from the earth's surface from escaping. But the amount of carbon dioxide and other insulating, or greenhouse, gases in the atmosphere is now rising fast, with potentially damaging effects on the earth's climate and on human health.

Carbon dioxide is produced by animals and plants and the burning of fossil fuels. Because trees fix carbon from the air, levels of carbon dioxide are also increased by deforestation. Each year 17 million hectares of tropical forest are being destroyed—an area the size of Austria.[2] In the past 100 years, since the beginning of the industrial revolution, the concentration of carbon dioxide in the atmosphere has increased by a quarter and is currently increasing at a rate of about 0·5% a year.[3] Concentrations are now higher than at any time in the past 160 000 years.[4] In 1988 human activity worldwide produced five billion tonnes of carbon, and the atmospheric concentration of carbon dioxide was estimated at 352 parts per million.[1] If in the next 100 years consumption of fossil fuels doubles—a conservative estimate—the concentration may rise to 600 parts per million: twice the level in 1850.[5]

In terms of sheer bulk atmospheric carbon dioxide is the main contributor to the greenhouse effect. But other gases present in the atmosphere—methane, nitrous oxide, and chlorofluorocarbons—are all more effective insulators, and their combined impact almost equals that of carbon dioxide (table).[6] Ozone, released at ground level as a result of the action of sunlight on urban air pollutants, also contributes to the greenhouse effect, as does water vapour.

The type and magnitude of changes that may result from the greenhouse effect are the subject of much controversy. In the past 100 years the earth's surface temperature has risen by an average of 0·6°C (figure). This could be a blip, but, according to proponents of the greenhouse theory, it is a sign that global warming is already occurring. Further increases of 2-5°C over the next 50 to 100 years have been predicted. This change is equivalent to the difference in temperature between the last ice age and now.[7]

Global warming could affect health both directly, by changing current patterns of disease, and indirectly, through its impact on sea

Concentrations, growth rates, atmospheric lifetimes and contributions to global warming of main greenhouse gases[8]

	Atmospheric concentration (parts per million)		Current rate of change/ year	Atmos-pheric life-time (years)	Contri-bution to global warming during 1980s (%)
	Pre-industrial (1750-1800)	1990			
Carbon dioxide	280	353	1·8 (0·5%)	50-200*	55
Methane	0·8	1·72	0·015 (0·9%)	10	15
Chlorofluorocarbon-11		280	9·5 (4%)	65	⎱ 17
Chlorofluorocarbon-12		484	17 (4%)	130	⎰
Nitrous oxide	0·288	0·31	0·8 (0·25%)	150	5

*The way in which carbon dioxide is absorbed by the oceans and biosphere is complex and a single value cannot be given.

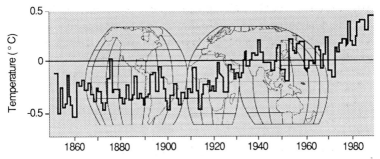

Changes in world temperatures in the past 140 years (0=1950-80 average).
Adapted from F Pearce[6a]

level and on the availability of agricultural land and water for
irrigation.[8]

Direct effects of global warming on health

People, especially those who are elderly, very young, or sick, are
not good at dealing with extremes of temperature. In temperate
climates the main concern is usually the effects of excessively cold
weather causing hypothermia and exacerbations of chronic lung
disease. But hot weather also holds its dangers. During heat waves
in Los Angeles the mortality is two to four times higher than normal,
and up to eight times normal in those aged over 85.[9] Mortality from
coronary heart disease and stroke increases when the average temperature exceeds 25°C,[10] and predictive models suggest that above
33°C mortality from all causes increases, mainly owing to deaths from
cardiovascular and respiratory disease. With a doubling of carbon
dioxide concentrations, the number of summer deaths in the United
States could increase sevenfold. Even taking into account acclima-
tisation and the likely reduction in winter deaths, models still predict
an overall increase in mortality (L S Kalkstein *et al*, international
conference on ozone modification and climate change, Washington,
DC, June 1986).

Changes in temperature and humidity could also mean the appear-
ance in temperate, industrialised countries of a number of diseases
that are currently limited to the tropics. The United States, for
example, could acquire mosquito borne diseases such as malaria,
dengue fever, arbovirus encephalitides, yellow fever, and Rift Valley
fever.[11]

21

Debate continues about whether the greenhouse effect will cause meteorological upset, leading to more storms and natural disasters.[12] If it does the world will have to contend not only with the immediate effects of death and disability but with the longer term sequelae of post-traumatic reactions, disabling psychiatric symptoms, and problems with psychological development in children.[8]

Indirect effects of global warming

The most easily comprehensible of the many potential consequences of global warming is the rise in sea level caused by the melting of glaciers and the polar ice caps. The size of this effect is controversial, and successive estimates have been increasingly conservative. In 1988, the talk was of a 6 m rise if the west Antarctic ice sheet were to melt.[13] In 1989 the United States Environmental Protection Agency predicted a rise of 0·5-2 m by 2100.[14] And in 1990 the International Panel on Climate Change estimated that during the next century the rise would not exceed 1 m.[15] This year the American National Academy of Sciences took an even more conservative line, estimating that an increase in temperature of 5°C would cause a maximum rise in sea level of 0·6 m.[3] This would be due mainly to thermal expansion because of increasing temperature and salinity. The academy con-

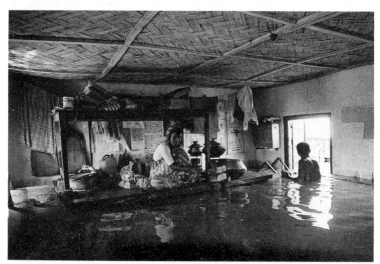

A quarter of Bangladesh could disappear underwater

cluded that substantial melting of the ice caps was unlikely but warned that unpredictable factors, such as the release of large amounts of methane from melting tundra, could have dramatic effects.

A rise in sea level of 1 m would mean the loss of large areas of inhabitable and agricultural land. One estimate puts the amount of land at risk from such a rise at 5 million km^2—an area comprising only about 3% of the earth's total land area but encompassing one third of the world's crop growing land and the homes of one billion people.[7] A 1 m rise in sea level would create 50 million environmental refugees—more than three times the number of all refugees today.[4] Low lying, densely populated areas would be most vulnerable. About a quarter of Bangladesh could disappear under water, displacing up to a third of the population, and the habitats of 46 million people living along the Nile and the Ganges are potentially threatened. America could lose more than 19 000 km of coastline around Florida and Miami, and areas of the Netherlands and the east coast of England could become submerged.

Water supplies from rivers and aquifers would become increasingly saline, and during the summer the amount and quality of available fresh water would fall. Changes in the patterns of rainfall could cause drought and desertification in currently fertile areas.

The predicted 20% increase in rain in winter and 5-10% reduction in summer would transform the grain belt in America's midwest— which provides 90% of the world's grain surplus—into desert.[12] A 2°C rise in temperature could mean a decline in the wheat yields of Europe and North America of between 3% and 17%.[16] Already in the past few years yields have fallen because of drought. In 1989 the world produced 18 million tons less grain than it consumed. An annual surplus of 28 million tons is needed to keep pace with population growth.[2] Overall temperature conditions necessary for productive agriculture would shift northwards, away from the middle of the United States and Europe into Canada and Siberia. But these areas may not have adequate rainfall or sufficiently fertile soil to allow equivalent productivity.

Crops are also damaged by excessive exposure to ultraviolet light and so the destruction of the ozone layer will reduce yields. Meanwhile, a high level of ozone at ground level, produced by the effects of sunlight on urban air pollutants, is also damaging. It is estimated to have caused the loss of up to 10% of crops in the United States during the 1980s.[17]

Countries in the developing world would suffer both the direct effects of drought and flood and the knock on effect of agricultural and economic decline in the West. The already present problems of feeding the world's growing population would be compounded by the increasing numbers of displaced people unable to grow their own food.

What should be done

The accumulation of greenhouse gases is largely the result of our dependence on fossil fuels for energy production. Nearly three quarters of Britain's carbon dioxide emissions result from the industrial and domestic burning of fossil fuels. A fifth comes from road traffic. Nitrous oxide and ozone are also products of fossil fuel consumption. Radical measures are needed to increase energy efficiency in power stations, industry, and homes to reduce the demand for fossil fuels. Governments should invest in alternative energy sources such as wind, wave, and solar power. But above all there is the need for traffic restraint. Industrial and domestic emissions in Britain have now stabilised, but by 2020 emissions of carbon dioxide will nearly double because of the continuing growth of road traffic. Policies for reducing the use of motor vehicles are discussed in a later chapter.

Efforts to stall and reverse deforestation are also important. Sustainable forestry policies should be adopted and the demand for timber reduced by changing building practices and reducing waste and inefficiency.

Carbon dioxide has a long half life: half of the carbon dioxide produced since the start of the industrial revolution remains in the atmosphere today.[5] Stabilising emissions is not the same as stabilising concentrations of gases in the atmosphere. The United States Environmental Protection Agency has estimated that to stabilise atmospheric concentrations of carbon dioxide, emissions will have to be cut by 50% to 80%.[18] Individual countries have responded to this with varying amounts of enthusiasm. The Netherlands is committed to a 20% reduction in emissions by 2000 and Germany to a 25% reduction by 2005. This may be increased to 30% as a result of policy changes since reunification. Britain has agreed only to stabilise emissions by 2005, and the United States and the Soviet Union have so far refused to agree to any limits at all.

Conclusion

Scientists are no longer asking whether global warming is taking place; the questions now are: To what extent? and How fast?[19] Predictions, however, are based on scientific theories and modelling and so remain controversial. But while the debate continues so does the potentially disastrous accumulation of greenhouse gases. As with acute medical emergencies there is no time to wait for the return of the investigations which would confirm the diagnosis. It is necessary to act on the balance of probabilities rather than waiting, like criminal lawyers, for all reasonable doubt to be removed. Global warming may prove to be this decade's scare story, though the weight of scientific evidence makes that unlikely, but the risks of drastic climatic change are too great to ignore.

1 McElroy MB. The challenge of global change. *Bulletin of the American Academy of Arts and Science* 1989;**42**:25-38.

2 Brown LR, ed. *State of the world 1991: a Worldwatch Institute report on progress toward a sustainable society.* London: Earthscans Publications, 1991.

3 National Academy of Sciences. *Policy implications of greenhouse warming.* Washington DC, National Academy Press 1991.

4 Brown LR, ed. *State of the world, 1989: a Worldwatch Institute report on progress toward a sustainable society.* New York: W W Norton, 1989.

5 Leaf A. Potential health effects of global climatic and environmental changes. *N Engl J Med* 1989;**321**:1577-83.

6 World Resources Institute. *World resources 1990-91.* New York: Basic Books, 1990:14.

6a Pearce F. Warmer winters fit greenhouse model. *New Scientist* 1991;Jan 19:20.

7 Brown LR, ed. *State of the world 1990: a Worldwatch Institute report on progress toward a sustainable society.* New York: W W Norton, 1990.

8 Haines A, Fuchs C. Potential impacts on health of atmospheric change. *J Public Health Med* 1991;**13**:69-80.

9 Oeschli FW, Buckley RW. Excess mortality associated with three Los Angeles September hot spells. *Environ Res* 1970;**3**:277-84.

10 Rogot E, Padgett SJ. Associations of coronary and stroke mortality with temperature and snowfall in selected areas of the United States, 1952-1966. *Am J Epidemiol* 1976;**103**:565-75.

11 Longstreth JA. Human health. In: Smith JB, Tirpak D, eds. *The potential effects of global climate change in the United States.* Washington, DC: Environmental Protection Agency, 1989.

12 Intergovernmental Panel on Climate Change. *Policymakers summary of the scientific assessment of climate change report to the IPCC from working group I, 1990.* Bracknell: Meteorological Office, 1990.

13 Hansen J, Fung I, Lasis A, Lebedeff S, Rind D, Ruedy R, *et al.* Predictions of near term climate evolution: what can we tell decision makers now? In: *Preparing for climate change: proceedings of the first North American conference on preparing for climate change: a cooperative approach, October, 1987.* Washington, DC: Government Institutes, 1988:35-47.

14 Titus JG. Sea level rise. In: Smith JB, Tripak D, eds. *The potential effects of global*

climate change in the United States. Washington, DC: Environmental Protection Agency, 1989.

15 Houghton JT, Jenkins GJ, Ephraums JJ. *Climate change: the IPCC scientific assessment*. Cambridge: Cambridge University Press, 1990.

16 Warrick RA, Gilford RM, Parry ML. CO_2 climate change and agriculture. In: Bolin B, Doos BR, Jager J, Warrick RA, eds. *The greenhouse effect, climatic change and ecosystems. SCOPE 29*. Chichester: Wiley, 1986.

17 MacKenzie JJ, El-Ashry MT. *Ill winds: airborne pollution's toll on trees and crops*. Washington, DC: World Resources Institute, 1988.

18 Environmental Protection Agency. *Policy options; conference statement. The changing atmosphere: implications for global security, Toronto, June 1988*. Washington, DC: EPA, 1988.

19 Intergovernmental Panel on Climate Change. *Climate change*. Cambridge: Cambridge University Press, 1990.

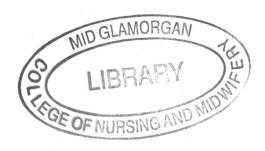

Dangers of ozone depletion

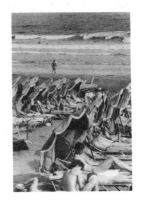

FIONA GODLEE

Atmospheric ozone absorbs ultraviolet light from the sun, especially in the ultraviolet range (260-320 nm), and protects plants and animals from its damaging effects. Loss of ozone from the earth's outer atmosphere could have dire consequences for human health.

Ozone is present in greatest abundance in the stratosphere (15-50 km above ground level.) In 1985 Joe Farman of the British Antarctic Survey reported considerable losses of ozone over the Antarctic during springtime. This confirmed fears first aired in the early 1970s that chlorofluorocarbons (CFCs), released into the atmosphere from aerosol sprays, light industry, and refrigeration, were destroying stratospheric ozone. Although less severe, depletion of ozone was also reported over the North Pole during the spring of 1989, and there is now evidence of generalised thinning of the ozone layer across the northern hemisphere. In 1988 the Ozone Trends Review Panel estimated a loss of 2-3% since the early 1970s at latitudes 53-64° north.[1]

Steady state concentrations of ozone in the stratosphere depend on the balance of the processes that form it and destroy it. Ozone is formed by the photochemical breakdown of molecules of oxygen. This occurs slowly and with a regeneration half time of three to four years. Chlorofluorocarbons are almost inactive at ground level, which allows them to rise unchanged into the stratosphere. There they generate free radicals which catalyse the photochemical breakdown of ozone. Chlorofluorocarbons have a long half life, persisting in the atmosphere for up to 100 years. Large amounts have been produced only since the second world war, and during the 1980s atmospheric concentrations were increased at a rate of about 5% a year.

An estimated 15% of the ozone layer over the Antarctic was

destroyed in the winter of 1989-90. Recently the National Aeronautics and Space Administration estimated a 4-5% loss of ozone over the northern hemisphere during the past decade.[2] Levels will continue to fall until well into the next century, possibly by as much as 20%. A 1% reduction in total column ozone is estimated to cause an increase in the amount of biologically effective ultraviolet B reaching the earth's surface of 1·5-2% (figure).[3]

Ozone depletion and health

The effects of ozone depletion on health are due mainly to the increased action of ultraviolet B on the skin and eyes (box). Sunburn and snow blindness result from acute exposure to intense sunlight. Long term exposure to the sun is associated with skin cancer and cataract formation.

The relation between exposure to the sun and skin cancer is well documented. Ultraviolet B falls within the photoabsorption spectrum of DNA and, when not eliminated by ozone in the stratosphere or melanin in the skin, it causes direct damage to DNA.

Non-melanocytic skin cancer

Both basal cell and squamous cell carcinomas are commoner in fair skinned people and are found on areas exposed to the sun for long

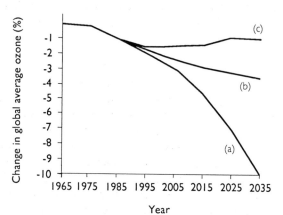

Global average changes in ozone concentrations for three patterns of chlorofluorocarbon use: (a) continuous growth; (b) 50% reduction by 1998; (c) replacement of halogenated chlorofluorocarbons by hydrochlorofluorocarbon 22. From Isaksen[3a]

Potential health effects of stratospheric ozone depletion[4]

Direct effects of ultraviolet B
Acute:
- Erythema (sunburn)
- Keratitis (snow blindness)

Chronic:
- Skin cancer
- Cataracts

Indirect effects of ultraviolet B
Decreased immune surveillance:
- Increased susceptibility to cutaneous infection
- Carcinogenesis

periods, particularly the head and neck. Incidences of both increase with age and with proximity to the equator and are higher in people who work outside such as farmers and fishermen.

In the United States there are currently an estimated 400 000 new cases of non-melanocytic skin cancer each year and 6000 deaths.[4] Among white Australians non-melanoyctic skin cancer is more than three times commoner than all other cancers combined. By the age of 75, two thirds of Australians will have been affected.[5] A report from the United Nations Environment Programme (UNEP) predicts that a 10% reduction in total column ozone would cause more than 300 000 additional cases of non-melanocytic skin cancer worldwide each year.[4a]

Malignant melanoma

Malignant melanoma is far less common than non-melanocytic skin cancer but it affects younger people and has a higher mortality. For this reason it has become an important public health issue.

Both genetic and environmental factors are important in the aetiology of malignant melanoma. As with non-melanocytic skin cancers, a relation exists between the incidence of cutaneous malignant melanoma and proximity to the equator. Malignant melanoma is commonest in fair skinned people who burn easily and in people in the higher socioeconomic groups. Short bursts of sunbathing—"flash frying"—are generally agreed to be more dangerous than exposure over prolonged periods. Australians have the highest incidence of malignant melanoma. In Queensland, Australia, the incidence is 10 times higher than in Britain and four times higher than in the United

States. About one in every 150 white male Queenslanders dies of malignant melanoma.

Attempts to predict the effect of ozone depletion on the incidence of malignant melanoma are more complicated and less reliable than for non-melanocytic skin cancers, but a 10% loss of ozone could increase mortality by up to 10% and incidence by as much as 20%.[6] The United Nations Environment Programme estimates that at least 4500 extra

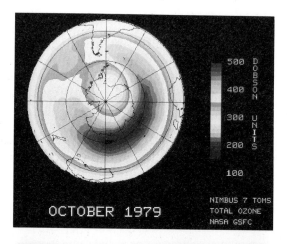

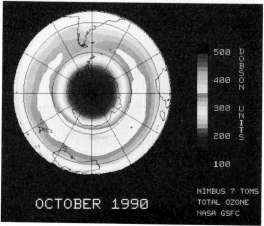

Satellite maps show worsening depletion of ozone layer over Antarctica between 1979, when the hole was first identified, and 1990

cases of malignant melanoma worldwide each year would result.[4a] Throughout the world the incidence of malignant melanoma is increasing and the age at diagnosis is falling.[7] However, publicity about the high mortality associated with malignant melanoma may persuade people to change their behaviour, resulting in less sun-bathing and a fall in package holidays to hotter areas.

Cataracts

The association with exposure to ultraviolet light is less clear for cataracts than for skin cancer. Senile cataracts are extremely common. In the United States they result in more than 600 000 operations each year. They are seen by some as the inevitable consequence of aging, but some evidence suggests that the incidence increases with decreasing latitude. In addition, cataracts can be induced experimentally by exposure to ultraviolet light, especially ultraviolet B and C. The United States Environmental Protection Agency has estimated that a 10% reduction in ozone by 2050 would cause over 600 000 additional cases of senile cataract in the existing population of America and 4·5 million additional cases in people born in the United States over the next 40 years.[8]

Immunosuppression

The immunosuppressant effect of ultraviolet B irradiation has been shown experimentally in mammals and could play a part in the development of cutaneous infections and skin cancer. Exposure to ultraviolet light may increase susceptibility to leishmaniasis and leprosy, and cold sores due to herpes simplex virus tend to be activated by sunlight.

Immunosuppression may indirectly increase the risk of skin cancer by reducing the body's immune surveillance. It is known that some skin cancers are commoner when the immune system is compromised by disease or drugs. In patients receiving immunosuppressive treatment after organ transplantation the incidence of squamous cell carcinoma may be 40 times higher than in controls.[9]

Urgent need for action

The need for action is urgent. The long residency time of chlorofluorocarbons in the atmosphere means that even if production is stopped completely their destructive effects will continue for many years. Since the Montreal accord in 1987, calling for a 50% cut in production by 1998, further progress has been made towards halting production of chlorofluorocarbons. In June 1990, 93 countries signed a United Nations agreement to stop producing chlorofluorocarbons by the end of the 1990s. Central to this agreement was the establishment of an international fund of $240 million to help countries in the Third World develop alternatives to chlorofluorocarbons.

Since then the date for a ban on chlorofluorocarbons has crept forward. The US government has committed itself to a ban on chlorofluorocarbons by the end of 1995, and Britain has promised to ban them by the beginning of 1996. Friends of the Earth believes that this is still not soon enough. "There are countries that have already stopped producing chlorofluorocarbons and halones," said a spokesman, Doug Parr. "In Germany it is illegal to use fresh halones—those that haven't come from recycling. It can be done. There are technological alternatives. We would say 'Do it now'."

On an individual level, skin cancer remains a preventable disease. Intensive education and publicity campaigns are needed, such as the successful "slip slop slap" campaign in Australia (slip on a shirt, slop on some sunscreen, and slap on a hat). People should be made aware of the risks of the sun and of ultraviolet tanning beds and should learn to recognise and look out for the early signs of skin cancer.

Conclusion

Ozone in the stratosphere shields us from the sun's damaging rays and is vital to life on earth. Unless its destruction is halted we can expect large increases in skin cancers and cataracts over the next few decades, not to mention widespread ecological changes. Doctors and other health professionals are in a position to influence both individual behaviour and government action, and they should work to avert this human and ecological catastrophe.

1 Watson RT. Present state of knowledge of the ozone layer. In: Russell Jones R, Wigley T, eds. *Ozone depletion: health and environmental consequences.* Chichester: Wiley, 1989, 51.
2 Kar RA. Ozone destruction worsens. *Science* 1991;252:204.
3 van der Leun JC. Experimental photocarcinogenesis. In: Russell Jones R, Wigley T, eds. *Ozone depletion: health and environmental consequences.* Chichester: Wiley, 1989.
3a Isaksen ISA. The beginnings of a problem. In: Russell Jones R, Wigley T, eds. *Ozone depletion: health and environmental consequences.* Chichester: Wiley, 1989:24.

4 Russell Jones R. Consequences for human health of stratospheric ozone depletion. In: Russell Jones R, Wigley T, eds. *Ozone depletion: health and environmental consequences.* Chichester: Wiley, 1989, 214.

4a UN Environment Programme. *Environmental effects of ozone depletion: 1991 update.* Nairobi: UNEP, 1992.

5 Giles G, Marks R, Foley P. Incidence of non-melanocytic skin cancer treated in Australia. *BMJ* 1988;**296**:13-7.

6 Elwood MJ. Epidemiology of melanoma: its relationship to ultraviolet radiation and ozone depletion. In: Russell Jones R, Wigley T, eds. *Ozone depletion: health and environmental consequences.* Chichester: Wiley, 1989, 179.

7 Jensen O, Bolander A. Trends in malignant melanoma of the skin. *World Health Stat Q* 1980;**33**:2-26.

8 Environmental Protection Agency. *Assessing the risks of trace gases that can modify the atmosphere.* Washington, DC: Environmental Protection Agency, 1987.

9 Shiel A. Cancer after transplantation. *World J Surg* 1986;**10**:389-96.

Waste disposal: fresh looks at a rotting problem

ALISON WALKER

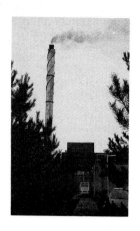

Most people take waste disposal for granted, yet it amounts to much more than the weekly collection of dustbin bags from our doorsteps. Britain alone produces more than 2·5 billion tonnes of waste a year from a wide range of sources including mines and quarries, factories, farms, hospitals, and construction sites (table). Historically, waste has not been disposed of with sufficient care and previous legislation has not been completely effective (box).

Air and water pollution, which to a large extent arise from waste discharged into the environment, are dealt with in other chapters in this book. The BMA's report *Hazardous Waste and Human Health* examines the effect of waste in greater detail.[2] This chapter considers certain aspects of waste of particular interest to the medical profession.

Clinical waste

Clinical waste arises from hospitals, health centres, general practitioners' and dentists' surgeries, veterinary surgeries, and from the homes of people with diseases such as diabetes or with renal failure who treat themselves. Among the potential risks from clinical waste, that from sharps (broken glass, needles, and other sharp instruments) is of considerable concern as a source of bloodborne disease agents such as hepatitis B virus and HIV. The risk of seroconversion after

Sources of waste, England and Wales

Type	Quantity (million tonnes/year)
Liquid industrial effluent	2000
Agriculture*	250
Mines and quarries (including china clay)*	130
Industrial	50
Hazardous and special	3·9
Special	1·5
Domestic and trade	28
Sewage and sludge	24
Power station ash	14
Blast furnace slag	6
Building	3
Medical wastes	0·15
Total	2505·15

*Not registered under Control of Pollution Act 1974.

percutaneous exposure to blood infected with HIV is only one in 200 but as high as one in five for hepatitis B virus. Immunisation against hepatitis B is available to all health workers, but no such precaution can be taken for HIV infection.[3]

Medical staff are not the only people at risk of sharps injuries in a hospital. During a 10 month study at a university hospital in the United States more than 320 sharps injuries were reported, of which 13% occurred during or after disposal; most of these injuries were caused by sharps protruding from rubbish waiting for disposal.[4] Another study, from the Hospital for Sick Children, Great Ormond Street, London, found that porters and those working in the central sterile supplies unit had the highest rate of sharps injuries.[5] At least 37 documented cases of seroconversion after occupational exposure to HIV have occurred world wide, most of which were caused by some form of sharps injury.[3] The only way to prevent transmission of infection is to assume that all clinical waste is potentially infected and adopt a universal safe practice.

Disposal of clinical waste

In Greater London alone some 30 000 tonnes of bagged clinical waste are produced every year.[6] The problem of disposing of such a large volume without risk is considerable.

Control of waste disposal

Specific waste disposal legislation in Britain is relatively recent but has taken several leaps forward since it was first introduced in the early 1970s. The first act aimed specifically at waste disposal was the 1972 Deposit of Poisonous Waste Act, passed after the discovery of drums of cyanide in a children's adventure playground in the Midlands.

The 1972 act was replaced by the more comprehensive Control of Pollution Act in 1974. This was criticised by the House of Commons Environment Committee in 1989.[1] According to the committee, the inadequacy of the regulations governing waste disposal had had serious consequences. Waste disposal authorities had acted as both poacher and gamekeeper —both operating and regulating waste disposal sites. Unscrupulous operators had been allowed "to dump waste, almost unchecked, because of variations in licensing and loopholes in the Control of Pollution Act 1974."

The 1990 Environmental Protection Act, the latest piece of legislation governing waste disposal in Britain, is intended to correct earlier deficiencies. One of its successes has been to separate out the roles of regulator and operator; regulation has become the sole responsibility of waste regulation authorities, policed by organisations such as Her Majesty's Inspectorate of Pollution and the National Rivers Authority, and disposal is carried out by waste disposal authorities and private contractors. An important theme of the Environmental Protection Act has been the control of waste from the "cradle to the grave."

The practice of segregating clinical waste from domestic and general waste by putting it into yellow bags and containers has been poorly adhered to according to evidence presented to the House of Commons environment committee.[1] This system was introduced in 1982 after concern was raised over the way in which clinical waste was being mixed with general waste. In the south east, in particular, clinical waste had been found in public areas, including holiday beaches. Even by 1989 the problem had not been solved. A scandal hit the headlines when clinical waste from London ended up on a landfill site licensed for domestic waste in Cheshire.

The London Waste Regulation Authority examined the disposal of clinical waste in 1989, taking evidence from both the public and private sectors.[6] It found many of the hospital incinerators to be old and overloaded, producing belching smoke and possibly dioxins, and operating below recommended temperatures—partly to economise on fuel. The authority also found scenes of burst yellow bags with their contents of dirty syringes and dressings spilling out on to the floor being handled by inexperienced disposal staff wearing minimal protective clothing. One of the authority's strongest recommendations was to reiterate the need for all clinical waste to be incinerated and not disposed of in landfill sites. For this to happen more incinerators would need to be built and existing ones brought up to standard. The BMA's report on hazardous waste echoed this response, adding that information on existing incinerators should be pooled.[2]

The lifting of crown immunity from clinical waste disposal in April 1991 allowed a welcome and long overdue review of the system. Hospitals now risk prosecution if they fail to meet the required standards under the Clean Air Act 1956 and 1968 and Control of Pollution Act 1974. Managers had until October 1991 to submit their programmes for upgrading but have until 1996 to implement the changes—far too long according to David Boyd of the National Association of Waste Disposal Contractors. The association has produced guidelines on clinical waste disposal covering segregation, packaging, transport, and disposal by high temperature incineration. "It's a professional game," said David Boyd, "which should not be carried out by untrained operators running aging inhouse incinerators." The standards defined in its guidelines, says the association, should be adopted by both private and hospital disposal teams.

Countries like Germany have introduced advanced systems for treating clinical waste at the site of production.[6] The waste is first shredded until it is unrecognisable and then treated with microwaves to ensure thermic disinfection. The waste can then be converted into granules if necessary and shipped to landfill sites. The new system can be used for treating all clinical waste including syringes, needles, and dialysis equipment, and other countries like Italy are already considering introducing it.

Waste from households, shops, and offices

The social reformer Edwin Chadwick, working during the nineteenth century, was one of the first people to link disease and death with poor sanitary conditions in the streets of Britain. Such conditions are now largely a thing of the past as local authority and private dustcarts regularly collect rubbish from households, shops, and offices. Thanks to this generally efficient service, very little harm actually comes from solid municipal waste. Problems can still arise when the waste is not collected during times of industrial action. A

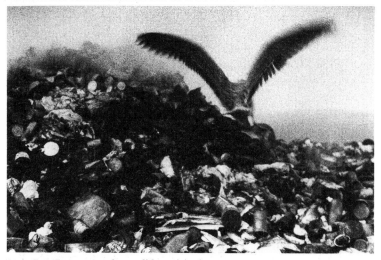

Very little harm comes from solid municipal waste

strike by refuse collectors in Liverpool during summer 1991 left rotting piles of rubbish on the streets, posing a health threat from the multiplying rat population, which acts as a reservoir for diseases such as leptospirosis.[7] Even without industrial action a health risk arises when unhygienic conditions allow cockroaches and fly populations to multiply among refuse since almost every known excreted pathogen has been isolated from these vectors.[8]

Fly tipping, or the illegal dumping of waste from both domestic and industrial sources, is a considerable problem in urban areas.[9] Far from being innocuous, fly tipped waste has been found to be "extremely hazardous," according to Mr Bill Townend of the London Waste Regulation Authority. A study carried out in London the 1980s, he said, found that 17 out of 58 sites of fly tipped material analysed were heavily contaminated with toxic substances such as heavy metals and posed a potentially serious risk to public health.

Hazardous industrial waste

Hazardous industrial waste has a high public profile and is therefore the main subject for public concern about safety of waste and its disposal. There have, however, been hardly any studies to provide scientific evidence to support this concern, and many of those existing are of poor quality.[2]

38

Tracing the cause of disease in an individual to previous exposure to a waste product is extremely difficult. Research based on exposure to waste products is limited, and many risk assessments are based on the known toxic effects of substances found in disposal sites, such as asbestos. This does not take into account the effects of mixing substances—the "cocktail compounds"—or the unknown nature of much waste material. Animal tests of toxicity have been used to study the effect of waste products in mammals, but they have limited application to humans. Though acute exposure to toxic substances may have clear cut effects, such as the respiratory and autonomic symptoms after poisoning with organophosphates, the effects of long term exposure are much more problematic and, with regard to public health, far more serious. Epidemiological studies may provide some of the answers but numerous confounding factors make the results difficult to interpret.

A Swedish study looked at the mortality among workers at a municipal waste incinerator.[10] Employment records dating back to 1951 were used to identify subjects for the study. More than 170 workers were identified who had been exposed to substances such as lead, mercury, cadmium, and carbon monoxide. An increased risk of lung cancer and ischaemic heart disease was found in the workers, thought to be caused by high occupational exposure to dust and gases at the incinerator. Although the study was criticised for being small, retrospective, and not fully adjusted for confounding factors, it is one of the few available on workers in the waste industry.

Extrapolating any results to the general population is fraught with problems. Toxic substances such as furans, dioxins, and polychlorinated biphenyls are ubiquitous in the environment and can make interpreting exposure difficult. Furthermore the technical means to detect trace amounts of many contaminants has outstripped the ability to predict their health risk.

Dioxin has become one of the more notorious toxic substances following the accident at a chemical plant at Seveso in Italy in 1976 when dioxins were released into the atmosphere. Dioxin is a generic term for 75 closely related compounds, the best known of which is 2,3,7,8-tetrachlorodibenzo-p-dioxin (TCDD). Dioxins are produced as a result of the combustion of organic material such as wood or the incomplete combustion of certain hazardous materials, including polychlorinated biphenyls. Experiments in animals have shown dioxins to be teratogenic and carcinogenic, but the results in humans are not as clear. A recent large study in the United States looked at

39

more than 5000 workers exposed to dioxins at 12 industrial plants.[11] The results overall were equivocal, but they did show a slight but significantly higher mortality from all cancers than expected—questioning the belief that low exposures are entirely safe.

Waste disposal sites

In Britain, about 90% of waste from factories, households, shops, and offices is taken to one of the 4000 or so controlled landfill sites for disposal. Most of the remainder is burned, either in a municipal incinerator or in one of the four specialised high temperature incinerators which deal with toxic waste. This contrasts with practice in many European countries—for example, Sweden—where some 60% of municipal waste is incinerated.

The transport and disposal of some toxic waste is carefully controlled under special waste regulations, which are part of the Control of Pollution Act 1974. The regulations cover the disposal of medicinal products available only on prescription, specified materials which are dangerous to human health, and substances with a flash point of 21 °C or less. Special documentation—a consignment note—is required so that the waste can be tracked from the premises of the waste producer to the point of final disposal.

Most people are suspicious of landfill sites and incineration plants which deal with waste. The NIMBY (not in my back yard) syndrome sums up most people's attitude towards them. A survey by the Department of the Environment in 1990 found the disposal of hazardous waste to be the public's biggest environmental concern—ranking higher than acid rain or pesticides.[12] "In the public mind it would appear that waste disposal sites are viewed as part of the problem of hazardous waste rather than as the solution," says the BMA in its review of hazardous waste and health.[2] But is the public right to be so concerned about waste disposal sites?

Landfill sites

Landfill sites present three potential hazards—ground water pollution, land contamination, and generation of explosive landfill gas. Contamination of ground water, when it occurs, presents a considerable problem since ground water is the source of about a third of the drinking water supply in England and Wales. Halogenated organic compounds, in particular, are very mobile in soils and can move into ground water easily. Traces have been found in many of the aquifers in Britain, especially those in old industrial regions. Modern industrial plants also threaten ground water supplies—for example, solvents from car manufacturing plants were found to be contaminating ground water in the West Midlands.[13] Legislation does exist to protect ground water. The European Community ground water directive, for example, restricts the level of substances allowed to be discharged into groundwater and these substances are monitored by the National Rivers Authority. Nevertheless, a study commissioned by the Department of the Environment in 1987 looked at 100 landfill sites in Britain and found that a third had caused contamination of ground or surface water.[14]

The health risks from low level contamination of water supplies are not fully known. Studies from the United States suggest that drinking private supplies from contaminated well water may be associated with an increase in the incidence of leukaemia, although these results have been disputed.[15] Public water supplies in Britain are better protected than private supplies from wells as they are regularly monitored and tested.

A combination of gases, particularly methane, can build up in a landfill site as landfill gas, with the potential to cause explosions with serious consequences. In 1986 gas escaped from an old landfill site leading to the explosion and destruction of a bungalow in Loscoe, Derbyshire. The Department of the Environment's review of 100 landfill sites found the problem of landfill gas to be seriously underestimated.[14] No gas control measures were found in 70% of sites and more than 50% lacked gas monitoring bore holes even though more than two thirds were within 500 metres of residential areas.

Contaminated land from previous indiscriminate dumping of toxic substances can have serious repercussions. Love Canal in Niagara City, New York, is a notorious example of this.[16] Between 1930 and 1952 about 20 000 tonnes of hazardous waste was dumped in the canal. It was subsequently filled in and built on. Twenty five years later tests were carried out in the area because foul smelling liquids and sludge had been found to be seeping into the basements of houses built on the site. Children were at particularly high risk because the school playground was built directly over the filled canal, and studies have suggested an association between living in Love Canal and short stature in children.[16]

Alternative waste disposal options

In countries like Sweden domestic waste recycling schemes flourish and bottle and can banks are a feature of most neighbourhoods. Britain has lagged behind in introducing these initiatives, but its new green policy spelt out in the Environmental Protection Act is intended to encourage waste minimisation and recycling both in industry and in the home. European commissioner for energy and the environment, Mr Stanley Clinton Davis, advised the House of Commons in 1989 that Britain ranked somewhere in the middle of the international hierarchy for adequate waste disposal practices.[1] It was joined by Belgium, France, Luxemburg, and Ireland. The best countries included Denmark and the Netherlands. Furthermore, the continued practice of codisposal (the joint disposal of industrial and household waste) in Britain has led others in Europe to believe that the British are sitting on a time bomb.

Conclusion

Recycling schemes aim at reducing the enormous volume of waste which needs to be disposed of every day. This should help prevent future waste disposal disasters like that at Love Canal, but the legacy of past bad practice and the continued mismanagement of landfill sites still present health hazards. Much more information is needed before health risks can be identified with certainty. As one official from the Department of the Environment said, "If you ask 12 doctors for advice on waste you are bound to get 13 different answers." Much more research needs to be done if the health risks of waste disposal are to be identified, and in time.

1 House of Commons Environment Committee. *Second report. Toxic waste.* London: HMSO, 1989.
2 British Medical Association. *Hazardous waste and human health.* Oxford: Waste Regulation Authority, 1989.
3 British Medical Association. *A code of practice for the safe use and disposal of sharps.* London: BMA, 1990.
4 Jagger J, Hunt EH, Brand-Elnaggar J, Pearson RD. Rates of needlestick injury caused by various devices in a university hospital. *N Engl J Med* 1988;**319**:284-8.
5 Waldron HA. Needlestick injuries in hospital staff. *BMJ* 1985;**290**:1285.
6 London Waste Working Party. *Clinical waste—an appraisal.* London: Oxford University Press, 1991.
7 Lowry S. Sanitation. *BMJ* 1990;**300**:177-9.
8 World Health Organisation. *Urban solid waste management.* Florence: World Health Organisation, 1991.
9 Royal Commission on Environmental Pollution. *Eleventh report, managing waste: the duty of care.* London: HMSO, 1985.
10 Gustavsson P. Mortality among workers at a municipal waste incinerator. *Am J Ind Med* 1989;**15**:245-53.

11 Fingerhut MA, Halperin WE, Marlow DA, Piacitelli LA, Honchal PA, Sweeney MH, *et al*. Cancer mortality in workers exposed to 2,3,7,8-tetrachlorodibenzo-*p*-dioxin. *N Engl J Med* 1991;**324**:212-8.

12 Central Statistical Office. *Social trends*. No 20. London: HMSO, 1990.

13 Department of the Environment. *Assessment of ground water quality in England and Wales*. London: HMSO, 1988.

14 Croft B, Campbell D. Characteristics of 100 UK landfill sites. In: *Proceedings of 1990 Harwell waste management symposium*. Harwell: United Kingdom Atomic Energy Authority, 1990.

15 Lagakos SW, *et al*. An analysis of contaminated well water and health effects in Woburn, Massachusetts. *Journal of the American Statistical Association* 1986;**81**: 583-6.

16 Paigen B, Goldman LR, Magnant MM, Highland JH, Steegman AT. Growth of children living near the hazardous waste site, Love Canal. *Hum Biol* 1987;**59**: 489-508.

Air pollution: I— from pea souper to photochemical smog

FIONA GODLEE

Air pollution has changed since the infamous winter fog of 1952 that killed 4000 Londoners.[1] Instead of the localised but lethal accumulation of sulphurous fumes—caused when large amounts of smoke from coal fires coincided with winter anticyclones (box)—the industrialised world now spends the summer draped in a photochemical haze of vehicle exhaust. Photochemical smog is, in its way, no less dangerous to health than the old winter fogs. There is increasing recognition of the role of smog in acute and chronic cardiorespiratory disease. But winter fogs, too, continue to take their toll. In the West clean air legislation has made them a thing of the past. But in eastern Europe and the Third World sulphurous pollution remains a major threat to health.

Sulphurous pollution

The World Health Organisation estimates that nearly 625 million people around the world are exposed to unhealthy levels of sulphur dioxide, and more than a billion people—one in five of the world's population—to excessive levels of particulate pollution.[2] Sulphur dioxide and particulates such as soot are the main airborne products from burning high sulphur fuel. Given the right meteorological

Winter fogs

The dangers of sulphurous pollution were most dramatically illustrated in December 1952 when a dense fog covered London killing up to 4000 people (fig 1). Other industrial cities had suffered similar, though less severe, episodes. Glasgow experienced two severe fogs in the winter of 1909, and another in 1925, all accompanied by an increase in mortality. In December 1930, five days of polluted fog killed more than 60 people in Belgium's industrial Meuse valley; and in Donora, Pennsylvania, 18 people died because of polluted fog during a two week period in October 1948.[1]

These pea souper fogs depended as much on meteorological conditions as on emissions of sulphur dioxide and soot. The anticyclone that settled over London on 5 December 1952 heralded a rare period of calm weather. Temperature inversion—a cold layer of air at ground level overlayed by a zone of warmer air—prevented the air from circulating and allowed the build up of emissions from low lying industrial and domestic chimneys. The trapped emissions combined with moisture in the cold air to form a deadly fog of acid vapour and black smoke.

Concentrations of sulphur dioxide reached a peak of nearly 4000 $\mu g/m^3$—more than 10 times the maximum level set down by the World Health Organisation as safe to breathe for one hour.[2] The victims—mostly young children and people over 65—died of heart and lung disease. In the week after the fog, sickness claims doubled and admissions to hospital rose from a daily average of 750 to 1110. Ammonia bottles with wicks brought the only relief from bronchial irritation, bronchospasm, dyspnoea, and cyanosis caused by the acidic air.

conditions—cold, moist air—and the presence of certain metal catalysts in polluted droplets of water—they combine to form aerosols of sulphuric acid. Easily inhaled into the lungs, this is probably the component of winter pollution that causes most damage to health.[3]

Pollution derived from high sulphur fuel has been linked with chronic bronchitis in adults and chest infections in children since the 1940s, though some studies have found no clear association.[4] In one study patients with bronchitis had significant exacerbations when concentrations of black smoke and sulphur dioxide in the air exceeded 250 $\mu g/m^3$ and 500 $\mu g/m^3$ respectively.[5] A study in Sheffield found an increase in both upper and lower respiratory tract infection in children living in heavily polluted areas.[6]

More recently, despite a fall in pollution from high sulphur fuels,[2]

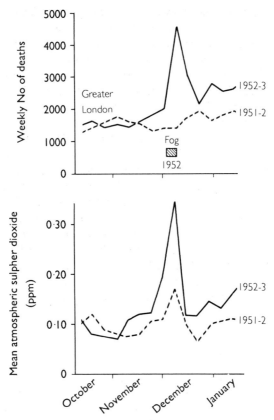

FIG 1—*Weekly number of deaths and atmospheric pollution in greater London, 1951-2 and 1952-3.*[1] [Conversion: 1 ppm=2860 $\mu g/m^3$ sulphur dioxide.]

studies in various countries have shown an association between acid aerosols and morbidity and mortality, especially among people with asthma (D V Bates, meeting of the British Thoracic Society, Birmingham, 13 July 1990). Outcome measures affected by concentrations of sulphur dioxide and sulphates include increased absenteeism from work,[7] respiratory symptoms in children,[8] lowered forced expiratory volume in one second,[9] increased emergency visits to hospital,[10] and increased prevalence of and mortality from asthma and bronchitis.[11-13]

The health effects of airborn particles—soot and other solids—are difficult to separate from those of other pollutants with which they are formed and with which they interact. Acid gases, for example, are adsorbed on to the surface of particulates and are carried into the lungs. The depth to which particles penetrate the respiratory tract depends on their size—smaller particles penetrating further—and the degree of mouth breathing. The depth of penetration is increased during exercise.[2] Clearance of particulate matter from the lungs is reduced in smokers and people with cystic fibrosis because of damage to the mucociliary system.

In the West pollution control has greatly reduced visible particulate pollution in air. But poor visibility at airports—an indication of levels of particles in air—has recently been linked with ill health. This has been attributed to fine airborne particles composed of sulphates.[14] But diesel fumes have now replaced coal burning as the major source of visible particulates in the West, being responsible for 90% of particulates in urban areas and one third of total emissions.[15] On the basis of occupational studies in people heavily exposed to diesel fumes, the International Agency for Research on Cancer concluded that diesel engine exhaust was "probably" carcinogenic to man.[16] I examine the possible relation between air pollution and cancer in the next chapter.

Clean Air Act 1956

The London fog of 1952 was sufficiently severe to force the British government to legislate. The 1956 Clean Air Act established smoke free zones in which only smokeless fuel, gas, or electricity could be used. This, combined with a fall in industrial pollution, has cut emissions of smoke in the United Kingdom by 85% over the past 30 years.[17] But Britain's success on the domestic front has been accompanied by poor performance internationally. The 1956 act also introduced the government's tall stack policy, now much criticised by environmental groups in Britain and Europe. Rather than requiring industry to reduce emissions, the policy ensured that pollutants were discharged from high chimney stacks to allow dispersal and dilution in the atmosphere. It put an end to winter smogs in Britain but has had catastrophic effects in Scandinavia, where acidic pollution from Britain falls as acid rain, damaging forests, crops, and aquatic life.

Other industrialised countries have also shifted from multiple small sources of pollution—such as domestic furnaces—to large single sources such as power stations, benefiting from improved air quality locally but contributing to the long distance effects of acid air pollution. They have, however, tended to combine tall stacks with strict limits on emissions. In the 1970s Japan, for example, installed scrubbers in its power stations to reduce emissions of acidic gases. Over a decade later Britain is following suit.

Developing disaster

In the floundering economies of the Third World and eastern Europe the poor quality of raw materials combined with inadequate pollution controls and reliance on poorly maintained diesel vehicles are wreaking havoc with the environment, recreating scenes from the early days of industrialisation in the West. Increasing urbanisation and the growing demand for energy can only make things worse. In China, for example, output of coal increased by more than 20 times between 1949 and 1982, and energy targets will mean a further doubling in the next decade.[18] In eastern Europe—where oil, natural gas, and hard coal have been scarce during the past 40 years—brown coal has formed the basis for industrial development. It has a high content of ash and sulphur and about half the energy value of hard coal, meaning that twice as much must be consumed to produce a given amount of energy.

Firm data on levels of air pollution in these countries are difficult to come by, but according to the World Health Organisation and the United Nations Environment Programme, during the 1980s annual average concentrations of particulate matter in New Delhi and Beijing were as much as five times the WHO standard.[2] In India emissions of sulphur dioxide have nearly tripled since the early 60s[18] and in Weimar in eastern Germany for the past three successive winters concentrations of sulphur dioxide have been higher than in London in December 1952 (H E Wichmann, personal communication) (fig 2).

The effects on health are predictable. In eastern Germany, for example, the mortality from bronchitis, asthma, and lung disease in men is reported to be the highest in Europe and double the European average. In parts of the southern industrial regions of eastern Germany life expectancy is from three to eight years below the national average and 90-100% of children have respiratory diseases. In the highly polluted industrial regions of Poland there are reports of increases in inflammation of the eyes and upper respiratory tract, in toxaemia (especially in children), and in illness related to tumours. In the lignite mining area in the north of Czechoslovakia the general sickness rate is two to 12 times higher than elsewhere in

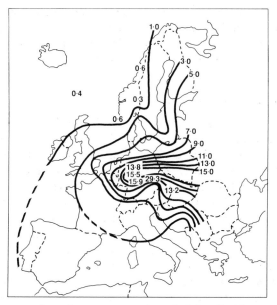

FIG 2 – *Annual mean concentrations of sulphur dioxide* *(μg/m³), 1985.*[19] [Conversion: *1 mg/m³=0·35 ppm* *sulphur dioxide.*]

the country, and children living there have an increased incidence of serious and complicated diseases of the upper respiratory tract. Allergic diseases in Czechoslovakian children increased 10-fold between 1962 and 1982, with a similar increase in congenital development defects and sight defects.[19]

These are broad brush strokes and many of the data are anecdotal. But one recent study attempted to link data on health with actual levels of pollution. It grouped over half a million 19 year old Polish army recruits according to the mean annual sulphur dioxide concentrations in the region of Poland from which they came. As the concentrations increased from fewer than 0·005 parts per million to more than 0·028 parts per million, the prevalence of chronic bronchitis increased more than threefold and that of asthma more than fivefold.[20]

The problems facing eastern Europe are considerable. The pace of change in 1989 and 1990, with the fall of the Berlin wall and the rapid improvement in East-West relations, has left an impression that similar rapid progress to a cleaner eastern Europe is simply a

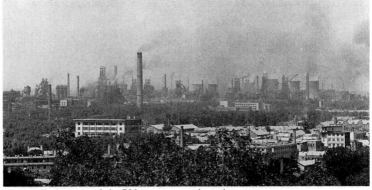

Poor pollution controls in China are recreating winter smogs

formality. But tens, and perhaps hundreds, of millions of pounds may be necessary to halt the deterioration and begin the cleaning up operation.[19] Confronted with other pressing demands on their limited finances, many of the countries in eastern Europe may allow the environment to slip down their list of priorities. Even within the environmental portfolio there are more urgent matters than air pollution. A meeting of eastern European and European environment ministers in Dublin in 1990 concluded that aging nuclear power stations and inadequate disposal of nuclear waste presented the most immediate threat to human health in eastern Europe.

Countries in eastern Europe and the developing world are confronted with a dilemma. Before they can make environmental issues a realistic priority, they need economic growth to support the necessary financial investment. But in the short term such growth will itself add to the problem of pollution. Environmental recovery will be achieved only at great financial cost and will require carefully coordinated aid and investment from the West.

There is, however, an up side to this grim scenario. Developing countries, behind as they are in the industrial race, now have the chance to learn from the mistakes of the West. This would mean not simply rerouting pollutants into the atmosphere but reducing their production, by both enforcing strict control of pollution at source and encouraging energy efficiency to cut demand. The increasing popularity of diesel vehicles, which produce large amounts of particulate matter, especially when poorly maintained, contributes to the problem of sooty smog in developing countries. Controlling emissions from road vehicles and discouraging the use of cars by providing adequate public transport would help reduce the environmental and human burden of airborne sulphur and soot.

Conclusion

Legislation in the West has been largely successful in bringing an end to winter smogs, but elsewhere in the world people are still suffering as a result of the uncontrolled burning of high sulphur fuel. Meanwhile, the West is experiencing problems of its own. The tall stack solution to winter fogs, coupled with the increase in road transport, has committed large areas of Europe and America to photochemical smog and acid rain. The health effects of these newer pollutants are only now being recognised. They are considered in the next chapter.

1 Ministry of Health. *Mortality and morbidity during the London fog of December 1952.* London: HMSO, 1954. (Reports on public health and medical subjects 95.)
2 World Health Organisation. *Air quality guidelines for Europe.* Copenhagen: WHO, 1987.
3 United Nations Environment Programme and World Health Organisation. *Assessment of urban air quality.* Nairobi: Global Environment Monitoring System, 1988.
4 Holland WW, Bennett AE, Cameron IR, Florey CV, Leeder SR, Schilling RS, *et al.* Health effects of particulate pollution: reappraising the evidence. *Am J Epidemiol* 1979;**110**:527-659.
5 Lawther PJ, Waller RE, Henderson M. Air pollution and exacerbations of bronchitis. *Thorax* 1970;**25**:525-39.
6 Lunn JE, Knowelden J, Handyside AJ. Patterns of respiratory illness in Sheffield infant school children. *Br J Prev Soc Med* 1967;**21**:7-16.
7 Ponka A. Absenteeism and respiratory disease among children and adults in Helsinki in relation to low level air pollution and temperature. *Environ Res* 1990;**52**:34-46.
8 Goren AI, Hellman S. Prevalence of respiratory symptoms and diseases in school children living in a polluted and in a low polluted area in Israel. *Environ Res* 1988;**45**:28-37.
9 Brunekreef B, Lumens M, Hoek G, Hofschreuder P, Fischer P, Biersteker K. Pulmonary function changes associated with an air pollution episode in January 1987. *Journal of the Air Pollution Control Association* 1989;**39**: 1444-7.
10 Bates DV, Baker-Anderson M, Sizto R. Asthma attack periodicity: a study of hospital emergency visits in Vancouver. *Environ Res* 1990;**51**:51-70.
11 Derriennic F, Richardson S, Mollie A, Lellouch J. Short term effects of sulphur dioxide pollution on mortality in two French cities. *Int J Epidemiol* 1989;**18**: 186-97.
12 Hatzakis A, Katsouyyanni K, Kalandidi A, Day N, Trichopoulos D. Short term effects of air pollution on mortality in Athens. *Int J Epidemiol* 1986;**15**:73-81.
13 Imai M, Yoshida K, Kitabatake M. Mortality from asthma and chronic bronchitis associated with changes in sulfur oxides air pollution. *Arch Environ Health* 1986;**41**:29-35.

51

14 Ostro BD, Rothschild S. Air pollution and acute respiratory morbidity: an observational study of multiple pollutants. *Environ Res* 1989;50:238-47.

15 Van den Hout KD, Rukeboer RC. *Diesel exhaust and air pollution. Research Institute for Road Vehicles.* Delft: Toegepast Natuurwetenschappelijk Onderzoek, 1986.

16 International Agency for Research on Cancer. *Diesel and gasolene engine exhausts and some nitroarenes.* Lyons: IARC, 1989. (Monographs on the evaluation of carcinogenic risk to humans, vol 46.)

17 Holman C. *Air pollution and health.* London: Friends of the Earth, 1989:1.

18 French HF. Clearing the air. In: Brown LR, ed. *State of the world 1990. A Worldwatch Institute report on progress towards a sustainable society.* New York: W W Norton, 1989:100.

19 Russell J. *Environmental issues in eastern Europe: setting an agenda.* London: Royal Institute of International Affairs and World Conservation Union, 1990.

20 Hertzman C. *Poland: health and environment in the context of socioeconomic decline.* Vancouver: Health Policy Research Unit, University of British Columbia, 1990. (Discussion paper 90, 2D.)

Air pollution: II—road traffic and modern industry

FIONA GODLEE

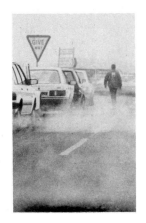

Summer smog is a cocktail of volatile hydrocarbons, oxides of nitrogen, sulphur dioxide, and carbon monoxide emitted from road vehicles, industry, and power stations. When acted on by sunlight it produces ozone, which is a potent respiratory irritant. At best photochemical smog is unpleasant, at worst it is harmful to health (table).

Ozone

Ozone at ground level builds up on sunny, still days when temperature inversion—a cold layer of air at ground level covered by a zone of warmer air—prevents the air from circulating. Concentrations reach a peak in the early afternoon and are often highest in rural areas. This is because anticyclones spread photochemical smog from cities, and rural areas lack nitric oxide, a constituent of urban pollution that scavenges ozone to form nitrogen dioxide and oxygen.

At low concentrations ozone causes coughing; nausea; irritation of the eyes, nose, and throat; and headaches. At higher concentrations, 150-200 parts per billion, it damages lung function. Laboratory studies have shown reversible reduction in forced vital capacity, forced expiratory volume, and peak expiratory flow rate in people

Effects of pollutants, World Health Organisation standards and when they're exceeded

	Airborne particulates	Sulphur dioxide	Nitrogen oxides	Carbon monoxide	Ozone	Benzene
Source	Diesel exhaust (90% in towns), coal burning	Fossil fuels, power stations (73%), diesel exhaust	Motor vehicles (45%), power stations (35%)	Incomplete combustion of fossil fuel, tobacco smoke	Photochemical reaction between nitrogen oxides and hydrocarbons	Emissions and evaporation from petrol engine. Highest at petrol stations and in cars
Health effects	Carry acidic gases and volatile hydrocarbons into lungs; may be carcinogenic	Causes bronchitis, and bronchospasm (especially in people with asthma)	Irritates respiratory tract	Reduces oxygen carrying capacity of blood; causes headaches; impairs concentration; exacerbates angina; can precipitate arrhythmias and cardiac arrest; can retard fetal growth	Causes coughing; impaired lung function; eye, nose, and throat irritation; headaches; aggravates asthma and bronchitis	Causes leukaemia
Environmental effects	Causes soiling of buildings, reduced visibility, odour	Main constituent of acid rain; damages plants and aquatic life	One third of acidity of rainfall	Oxidises to carbon dioxide, contributing to greenhouse effect	Greenhouse gas; damages crops, trees, plastics, rubber, and paints	
WHO standard: 1 h average		150 µg/m³	400 µg/m³	30 mg/m³	76–100 ppb (150–200 µg/m³)	No safe level because carcinogenic
8 h average				10 mg/m³	50–60 ppb (100–120 µg/m³)	
24 h average	120 µg/m³	125 µg/m³	150 µg/m³			
1 yr average		50 µg/m³				
When exceeded	Regularly	1 h average regularly in London and throughout Britain	Busy roadside locations	8 h guideline exceeded 24 days in winter 1988 at one London site	Several times during summer 1989; one site in Devon reached 135 ppb	

Source: *Air Quality Briefing Sheet*. Friends of the Earth, 1991. [*Conversions*—sulphur dioxide: 1 ppm=2860 µg/m³, 1 mg/m³, 1 mg/m³=0·35 ppm; nitrogen dioxide: 1 ppm=1880 µg/m³, 1 µg/m³, 1 µg/m³=5·32×10⁻⁴ ppm; carbon monoxide: 1 ppm=1·145 mg/m³, 1 µg/m³=0·873 ppm; ozone: 1 ppm=2 µg/m³, 1 µg/m³=0·5 ppm.]

with asthma and in healthy volunteers.[1] The effects of ozone are worsened by exercise and prolonged exposure, although tolerance seems to occur after a few days. Ozone may also increase the susceptibility of people with asthma to common allergens.[2]

The link between ambient ozone concentrations and impaired lung function has been shown by studies on children in summer camps in the United States. Children had reduced forced vital capacity, forced expiratory volume, and peak expiratory flow rate when ozone concentrations rose during hazy weather. Lung function in children is affected to the same extent as in adults but children develop fewer symptoms and so are less aware of respiratory irritation.[3]

Chronic exposure to ozone may cause structural damage to the lungs. A pathologist in Los Angeles found that 29 out of 107 healthy teenagers who died in road accidents or of other non-respiratory causes had severe respiratory bronchiolitis of the type found in young smokers and in monkeys chronically exposed to high concentrations of ozone. (R P Sherwin, V Richters. Centriacinar region disease in the lungs of young adults. Meeting of the AWMA, Los Angeles, March 1990.) A further 51 teenagers had moderate changes.

No legislation controlling ozone concentrations in air exists in the United Kingdom or European Community, and guidelines from the World Health Organisation for peak ozone concentrations leave little or no safety margin. The guidelines are regularly exceeded in Britain during the summer, with ozone reaching concentrations known to cause acute symptoms and long term structural damage.

Asthma and allergy

Between 1971 and 1981 the number of people attending general practitioners' surgeries with asthma and hay fever doubled despite a fall in concentrations of grass pollen in the air. Read has summarised the evidence linking asthma and allergic disease with air pollution and concludes that "pollutants derived from traffic exhaust may exacerbate, and in some cases even initiate, both conditions."[2] But air pollution is not the only possible explanation for the rising toll from asthma; more inclusive diagnostic criteria, inadequate management, and side effects of drug treatments are alternative explanations.

Several constituents of air pollution cause bronchospasm in people with mild asthma and, at higher doses, in non-asthmatic people. Sulphur dioxide, for example, provokes asthma in susceptible people at 200 parts per billion,[4] a concentration which exceeds the one hour average concentration recommended in the WHO guidelines and which is regularly found in Britain. People with asthma also seem particularly susceptible to nitrogen oxides and acid aerosols.[5] In contrast, ozone impairs lung function equally in people with and without asthma, though it also sensitises people with asthma to other pollutants such as sulphur dioxide as well as to common allergens.[6]

Air pollution has increased over the past 40 years and so have admissions to hospital and deaths associated with asthma. Asthma was rare in Britain until after the first world war but the prevalence rose dramatically after the second world war. Rates of hospital admission for children with asthma trebled between 1959 and 1973,[7] and over the past 10 years Australia, France, England and Wales, Canada, and the United States have recorded an increase in deaths from asthma in the 5-34 year age group of 30% to 60%. (M Sears, world conference of lung health, Boston, Masachussetts, 1990.) Whether this is because of an increase in severity or in prevalence of asthma remains debatable.

Epidemiologists studying asthma face several difficulties. Potential confounding factors include idiosyncratic responses to allergens, smoking, and infectious agents and the effects of the weather on both the disease and levels of pollution. Added to these are the difficulty of relating levels of pollutants recorded at monitoring stations with actual levels experienced by individuals and the lack of universal criteria for diagnosing asthma.

But studies of major episodes of air pollution have shown an increase in new cases of asthma and in attack rates among people known to have asthma. Examples are studies of American army staff in Tokyo in the 1940s,[8] and of episodes during the middle of this century in the Meuse Valley, Belgium, Donora in Pennsylvania, and London. Since then several studies have found associations between local levels of pollutants, mainly sulphur dioxide and photochemical smog, and rates of asthma attacks and hospital admissions.[2]

Concentrations of pollutants in the environment rarely reach those required in laboratory studies to induce asthma, but a Spanish study suggests that pollutants act synergistically with allergens so that even low levels can cause bronchospasm.[9] Japanese studies have linked the prevalence of allergic rhinitis with particulate pollution from diesel engines, and in Britain air pollution has been shown to add to the effect of pollen in causing symptoms of hay fever.[10]

Cancer and air pollution

There is continuing controversy over the extent to which urban air pollution causes cancer. "In murder mysteries," says Dr Simon Wolff, a toxicologist at University College, London, "one often finds a corpse but no smoking gun. But when looking for specific evidence of the health impact of transport . . . there are a lot of smoking guns but apparently no corpses." Much research has been done, he says, on the risks of lung cancer from passive smoking and domestic radon, but there are few studies on the relation between traffic pollution and cancer. These studies, he says, show that exhaust fumes represent a risk for many different cancers far outweighing the small effects linked with passive smoking, radon, or diet.

Sir Richard Doll, professor of epidemiology in Oxford, disagrees. "In 1948 when we started working on trying to explain the increased incidence of cancer, air pollution was the favoured explanation," he said. "Most of us thought the rise in cancer was due to motor traffic. But the more work that has been done, the less connection is found." He acknowledges the small increase in risk of cancer that has been shown in some occupational groups such as engine and truck drivers but has not seen this reflected in population based data. "Its not a very popular thing to say these days, because nobody believes it," he said. "But there is no demonstrable relationship between air pollution and cancer." He believes that this does not rule out the possibility of an environmental risk too small to be detected.

In 1988 a working party for the International Agency for Research on Cancer concluded that diesel engine exhaust is "probably" and petrol engine exhaust "possibly" carcinogenic to humans.[11] This conclusion is based mainly on occupational studies, which use a person's job as a surrogate measure for their individual exposure to pollutants. Jobs producing high exposure to diesel exhaust include work on the railway, in bus garages, and as truck drivers, while petrol exhaust exposure is high among traffic control workers and professional drivers. Some studies have shown no excess risk of cancer, or a non-significant increase in risk, in these occupational groups.[12 13] Other studies have, however, found a small but significant excess risk of cancer, especially of the lung and bladder.

Garshick *et al* examined 19 396 deaths among a cohort of middle aged railway workers,[14] and found more deaths from lung cancer among workers regularly exposed to diesel exhaust than among those with no exposure. The excess risk was small but statistically significant and increased with duration of exposure. In another American study 1256 railroad workers who died of primary lung cancer were matched with two controls by age and date of death.[15] The study found a significantly increased risk of lung cancer (odds ratio 1·4; 95% confidence interval 1·1 to 1·9) in those aged 64 or less who had been exposed to diesel exhaust for 20 years. No such effect was found in the older age group, but many of these had retired before the large scale introduction of diesel engines to the railways.

Jensen *et al* found a significant excess risk for bladder cancer among land transport workers and bus, taxi, and truck drivers in Denmark.[16] The excess risk increased with exposure for all except land transport workers. Steenland *et al* found a significant increase in the incidence of bladder cancer in men from Ohio with more than 20 years' employment as truck drivers (odds ratio 12·0; 95% confidence interval 2·3 to 62·9) and railroad workers (2·2; 1·2 to 4·0).[17]

The children of adults exposed to engine exhaust may have increased risks of cancer. Possible mechanisms are mutation of germ cells, intrauterine exposure, or early postnatal exposure. One study found that children of car mechanics and service station attendants had a non-significant increase in leukaemia, lymphoma, and neurological cancer and a small but significant increase in cancer of the urinary tract (odds ratio 2·9; 1·0 to 8·1). No increase in any forms of cancer was found in children of motor vehicle drivers.[18] In contrast, a Finnish study showed a significant increase in cancer among the children of professional drivers (odds ratio 1·9; 1·1 to 3·7).[19]

There are problems with all of these studies. The most important one is that engine exhaust is ubiquitous in urban areas: there is therefore no such thing as an unexposed control group. There is also the "healthy worker effect"—people in regular employment tend to have lower than average mortality. Both of these problems will tend to cause underestimation of the risks. Factors likely to exaggerate or simply misrepresent the risks are smoking, passive smoking, and exposure to asbestos, and the use of job histories as surrogate measures of exposure.

The difficulty of showing any excess risk in people exposed to high levels of pollution through their work makes it unlikely that studies of the general population exposed to much lower levels of pollution would show any excess risk of cancer. Studies apparently showing this have, however, been published. An American case control study of 328 children with cancer found that children living in areas of high traffic density (500 or more vehicles a day) had an excess risk of developing cancer in general (odds ratio 1·7; 1·0 to 2·8) and leukaemia in particular (2·1; 1·1 to 4·0).[20] The study has, however, been criticised because of inappropriate controls, and is, according to Richard Doll, "uninterpretable." Another study showed an increase in the overall incidence of cancer in a Swiss mountain valley after a motorway was built and correlated the local increase in cancer and levels of polyaromatic hydrocarbons in the soil.[21] It is, however, confounded by the increase in cancer throughout Switzerland.

In conclusion, people heavily exposed to diesel and petrol exhaust are at increased risk of developing cancer, especially of the lung and bladder, but the risks are small. Whether the general population is at risk of cancer from air pollution remains questionable, but any such risk is likely to be extremely small. Whether petrol or diesel is the most environmentally friendly fuel remains open to debate (box).

Benzene

One particular component of petrol, benzene, deserves special comment. Benzene is a volatile hydrocarbon also present in cigarette smoke and some domestic solvents and causes leukaemia in man.[25] The main source of benzene in air is emission from petrol engines and evaporative loss during handling, distribution, and storage of petrol. Levels of airborne benzene are closely related to traffic density and range from one to 50 parts per billion. But benzene also builds up

---

Diesel or petrol—which is more environmentally friendly?

Diesel engines burn fuel more efficiently than conventional spark ignition petrol engines and emit fewer hydrocarbons and less carbon monoxide. The lower ignition temperatures required also result in fewer oxides of nitrogen. Higher fuel efficiency means diesel engines emit about 18% less carbon dioxide per kilometre.[22] Energy savings also occur at the refinery since diesel requires less processing than petrol.

The main disadvantage of diesel engines is their emission of sulphur dioxide and particulate pollution —the major components of winter pollution. The popularity of diesel vehicles is adding to sulphurous pollution from other sources in the developing world and threatens to reintroduce sooty smogs to urban areas in the West, where diesel fumes are now responsible for 90% of airborne particulate matter.[23] Diesel engines emit about 10 times more particulate pollution than conventional petrol engines and 30-70 times more than petrol engines fitted with catalytic converters.[24] Diesel vehicles are also noisier.

inside cars, reaching concentrations close to the limit for occupational exposure in America.[26] The World Health Organisation insists that there is no safe level of benzene because of its known ability to cause cancer.

Extrapolation of the risks of environmental exposure to benzene from data on high dose is speculative, but WHO guidelines estimate that the lifetime risk of leukaemia at benzene concentrations of 0·3 parts per billion is four cases per million people. The California Air Resource Board has estimated that the added lifetime risk of developing leukaemia from exposure to benzene in Los Angeles is 101 to 780 cases per million people.[27]

Pollution control

Strategies to reduce photochemical smog must reduce both stationary and mobile sources of pollution. Substantial progress has been made in reducing emissions from power stations in the past 20 years, but many obstacles still remain. Electrostatic precipitators and filters can reduce particulate emissions by 99·5% and are now mandatory in almost all countries in the Organisation for Economic Cooperation and Development. But they have no effect on particulates of sulphates and nitrates formed from gaseous emissions outside the chimney stack. Though not as visible in the air as particles of soot, these cause damage to the lungs.[28]

Emissions of sulphates can be reduced by scrubbers, which reduce emissions of sulphur dioxide from individual power stations by as much as 95%. They are fitted only to newer power stations. Reducing emissions of nitrates is more difficult. Selective catalysts can reduce emissions of oxides of nitrogen by 80-90%, but they are expensive and are in widespread use only in Japan. Elsewhere in the world, various forms of modified combustion are used which reduce emissions by only 30-50%.

In the West new power stations must now conform to strict regulations for pollution control. But controlling emissions from existing plants means fitting the devices retroactively, and only Britain, the Netherlands, Scandinavia, and Germany have undertaken this on any scale.

Like the tall stack policy of the 1950s and 1960s, which cured the winter fogs but caused far flung problems with acid rain, these strategies create problems of their own. For example, desulphurising emissions from power stations produces large amounts of hazardous ash. The strategies also have no effect on emissions of carbon dioxide—the main greenhouse gas.

Emissions of carbon dioxide from domestic and industrial combustion in Britain have now stabilised because of energy efficiency measures, and in the next 10 years further reductions in emissions of nitrogen oxides and sulphur dioxide will be required to conform with European Community directives on large combustion plants. But these improvements will have little impact on overall emissions of pollutants, a growing proportion of which come from road transport.

Technical fixes for road traffic emissions

Road traffic emits a fifth of carbon dioxide, a third of airborne particulates and volatile organic compounds, half of oxides of nitrogen, and almost all carbon monoxide in the air. Attempts to reduce this pollution involve various technical fixes such as catalytic converters and filter traps. A European Community directive will enforce the fitting of catalytic converters to all new cars by 1993 and of particulate traps to all new trucks and buses by 1996. Environmental groups are now calling for the compulsory fitting of similar devices to existing vehicles.

Oxidation catalysts convert hydrocarbons and carbon monoxide into carbon dioxide and water. But they have no effect on oxides of nitrogen and as a result have been largely superceded by three way catalytic converters. These reduce emissions of carbon monoxide by 80%, hydrocarbons by 90%, and oxides of nitrogen by 95%.[29]

One of the unforeseen advantages of catalytic converters is that they can work only with lead free fuel. Their widespread introduction in America and Japan, prompted by the need to reduce photochemical smog, has therefore dramatically reduced the amount of lead in air (figure). In America, lead in air fell by 96% between 1970 and 1987, and average blood levels fell by more than one third between 1976 and 1980.[31]

But catalytic converters also have disadvantages,[22] and they have no effect on emissions of carbon dioxide from cars. Because of their adverse effect on fuel economy—reducing it by 1-10%[32]—they may even increase emissions of carbon dioxide. They begin to act only when the engine has warmed up, and most journeys are short and do not allow the engine to warm up sufficiently.

Neither oxidation nor three way catalytic converters are compatible with diesel engines. Pollution from diesel vehicles is being tackled by

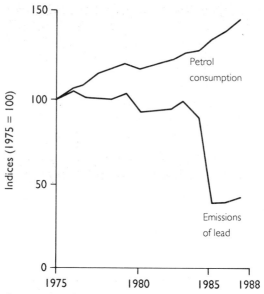

*Consumption of petrol and emissions of lead from road
vehicles with petrol engines, United Kingdom*[30]

improved engine design—such as turbo charging which makes use
of the exhaust fumes—and particulate traps, which may reduce particulate emissions by up to 85%.

The main source of benzene is evaporative emission, and carbon
cannisters to reduce evaporative emissions at refueling sites are being
considered by the British government. Vapour retrieval systems are
already compulsory in California. Reducing the amount of benzene in
petrol would, however, be impractical, according to the Department
of Transport and would increase the amount of carbon dioxide
produced.

Technical fixes have their limits. They can reduce emissions from
each vehicle and so reduce the amount of pollution produced per
kilometre travelled. In the short term this will reduce overall emissions, but the effect will soon be swamped by the growth in the
number of vehicles. The Department of Transport estimates that by
2025 vehicle miles travelled in the United Kingdom will double.
Catalytic converters will cause a fall in emissions of oxides of nitrogen
from their current level in Britain of 1·3 million tonnes, but by 2020
emissions will be back up to 1·38 million tonnes and rising.[33]

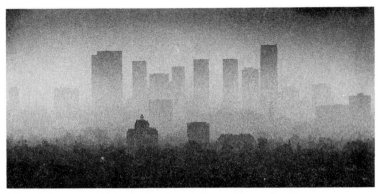

The only long term solution to summer smog is to reduce road traffic

Conclusion

Photochemical smog is dangerous to health. The contribution from stationary sources of pollution—power stations and industry—is shrinking. Further reductions could result from investing in energy efficiency programmes and transferring to alternative energy sources like wind, wave, and solar power. But attempts to reduce mobile sources of pollution through technical fixes will be effective only in the short term. The only effective long term solution to modern air pollution is to reduce road traffic.

1 World Health Organisation. *Air quality guidelines.* Copenhagen: WHO, 1987.

2 Read C. *Air pollution and child health.* London: Greenpeace, 1991.

3 Avol EL, Linn SW, Shamoo DA, Valeria LM, Anzar WT, Venet TG, *et al.* Respiratory effects of photochemical oxidant air pollution in exercising adolescents. *Am Rev Respir Dis* 1985;**132**:619-22.

4 Linn WS. Respiratory effects of sulphur dioxide in freely breathing, heavily exercising asthmatics: a dose response study. *Am Rev Respir Dis* 1983;**127**:234-9.

5 Mohsenin V. Airway response to nitrogen dioxide in asthmatic subjects. *J Toxicol Environ Health* 1987;**22**:371-80.

6 Koenig JQ. Prior exposure to ozone potentiates subsequent response to sulphur dioxide in adolescent subjects. *Am Rev Respir Dis* 1990;**141**:377-80.

7 Anderson HR. Increase in hospitalisation for childhood asthma. *Arch Dis Child* 1987;**53**:295-300.

8 Huber TE. New environmental respiratory disease (Yokohama asthma). *Archives of Industrial Hygiene and Occupational Medicine* 1954;**10**:399-408.

9 Berciano FA, Dominguez J, Alvarez FV. Influence of air pollution on intrinsic childhood asthma. *Ann Allergy* 1989;**62**:135-41.

10 Gunner G, Riley GA, Fitzharns P, Ashmore MR. Effect of air pollutants on hay fevery symptom severity [abstract]. *J Allerg Clin Immunol* 1991;**87**:185.

11 International Agency for Research on Cancer. *Diesel and gasoline engine exhausts and some nitroarenes.* Lyons: IARC, 1988. (IARC monographs on the evaluation of carcinogenic risk to humans. Vol 46.)

12 Kaplan I. Relationship of noxious gases to carcinoma of the lung in railroad workers. *JAMA* 1959;**171**:97-101.

13 Williams RR, Stegens NL, Goldsmith JR. Associations of cancer site and type with occupation and industry from the third national cancer survey interview. *J Natl Cancer Inst* 1977;**59**:1147-85.

14 Garshick E, Schenker MB, Munoz A, Segal M, Smith TJ, Woskie SR, *et al.* A retrospective cohort study of lung cancer and diesel exhaust exposure in railroad workers. *Am Rev Respir Dis* 1988;**137**:820-5.

15 Garshick E, Schenker MB, Mūnoz A, Segal M, Smith TJ, Woskie SR, *et al.* A case-control study of lung cancer and diesel exhaust exposure in railroad workers. *Am Rev Respir Dis* 1987;**135**:1242-8.

16 Jensen OM, Wahrendorf J, Knudsen JB, Sorensen BL. The Copenhagen case reference study on bladder cancer. Risks among drivers, painters, and certain other occupations. *Scand J Work Environ Health* 1987;**13**:129-43.

17 Steenland K, Burnett C, Osorio AM. A case-control study of bladder cancer using city directories as a source of occupational data. *Am J Epidemiol* 1987;**126**: 247-57.

18 Kwa SL, Fine LJ. The association between parental occupation and childhood malignancy. *J Occup Med* 1980;**22**:792-4.

19 Hemminki K, Saloniemi I, Salonen T, Partanen T, Vainio H. Childhood cancer and parental occupation in Finland. *J Epidemiol Community Health* 1981;**35**:11-5.

20 Savitz D, Feingold L. Association of childhood cancer with residential traffic density. *Scand J Work Environ Health* 1989;**15**:360-3.

21 Blumer M, Blumer W, Reich T. Polyaromatic hydrocarbons in soils of a mountain valley: correlation with highway traffic and cancer incidence. *Environmental Science and Technology* 1977;**11**:1082-6.

22 Howard D. *Energy, transport, and the environment.* London: Transnet, 1990.

23 Van den Hout KD, Rukeboer RC. *Diesel exhaust and air pollution.* Delft: Research Institute for Road Vehicles, 1986.

24 Organisation for Economic Cooperation and Development. *Transport and the environment.* Paris: OECD, 1988.

25 International Agency for Research on Cancer. Benzene and annex. In: *Some industrial chemicals and dyestuffs.* Lyons: IARC, 1982. (IARC monographs on the evaluation of the carcinogenic risk of chemicals to humans. Vol 29.)

26 Gilks JML, Boelsma van Houte E, Eyres AR, Rousseaux G, Roythorne C, Stanton DW, *et al. Health risk of exposure to non occupational sources of benzene.* Netherlands: The Hague, 1989. (CONCAWE report No 8/89.)

27 California Air Resource Board. *Report to the scientific review panel on benzene.* Los Angeles: Department of Health Services, 1984.

28 Ostro BD, Rothschild S. Air pollution and acute respiratory morbidity: an observational study of multiple pollutants. *Environ Res* 1989;**50**:238-47.

29 Holman C, Fergusson M, Robertson T. *The route ahead: vehicle pollution—causes, effects, answers?* London: World Wildlife Fund, 1990.

30 Central Statistical Office. Transport and the environment. *Social Trends* 1991;**20**: 147.

31 Brown LR. *State of the world 1990.* New York: W W Norton, 1990:103.

32 Organisation for Economic Cooperation and Development. *Energy and cleaner air: costs of reducing emissions.* Paris: OECD, 1987.

33 Fergusson M, Holman C, Barrett M. *Atmospheric emissions from the use of transport in the UK.* Vol 1. *The estimation of current and future emissions.* London: World Wildlife Fund/World Resources Research, 1989.

Transport: a public health issue

FIONA GODLEE

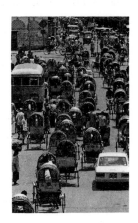

Most people will never own a car. But throughout the world cars continue to dictate transport policy. The growth in the world's car fleet—it now stands at 400 million—is whittling away the benefits of car ownership as machines built for speed are forced to idle in gridlocked cities. The problems caused by overdependence on private cars are now being recognised. The motor industry may be persuaded to tackle air pollution, but greener cars hold no answers for the other by blows of the motor car—traffic congestion, noise, road accidents, and social inequality.

Accidents

Road accidents are the most direct means by which transport affects health. In 1988 they caused more than 250 000 deaths worldwide. The dangers are greatest in the Third World, where roads carry a mixture of motorised and non-motorised vehicles—rickshaws, bicycles, carts—often unregulated and travelling at high speeds. Deaths from accidents are 20 times higher there than in the industrialised world.[1]

More than four fifths of all road accidents in Britain involve cars. But improvements in design have meant that travelling in a car is getting safer all the time. Since 1972 deaths among car occupants have halved. Meanwhile life for pedestrians and cyclists is becoming more hazardous. Britain has the highest child pedestrian mortality of any country in Europe. 1988 saw over 400 deaths in children aged 14 or less. In terms of years of life lost below the age of 70, road accidents, with their high proportion of young victims, are on a par with carcinoma of the lung, trachea, and bronchus. From 1952 to 1987 deaths among cyclists fell by two thirds, but taking into account the reduction in cycling the number of deaths per billion kilometres travelled almost doubled.[2]

Safety on the roads, or lack of it, is not necessarily reflected in accident statistics as people change their behaviour in response to perceived dangers. This so called risk compensation reduces the accident toll but has its own effects on people's lives. Warning children not to play on the streets, penning people in with guard rails, and redirecting them down pedestrian subways are all examples of risk compensation. They concentrate on removing pedestrians, especially children, from the danger instead of reducing the danger itself. No change in behaviour is asked of the motorist.[3] Risk compensation may take the form of avoiding certain types of transport. London has about 400 000 regular cyclists. The London Cycling Campaign estimates that another million people would cycle but are put off by the thought of accidents and air pollution.

Cycling helmets provide another form of risk compensation. Whether or not they are effective protection remains debatable. Those who wear them have reduced incidence and severity of head injury,[4] but this may be because they are generally more cautious. Liz Marriot of the London Cycling Campaign thinks that helmets do help, if only because they make the cyclist more visible to motorists, but they are of little benefit in high speed crashes. "They are made out to be the answer to cycling injuries. That's nonsense. It's not the cyclists that cause the problem."

Too many cars

The problem for cyclists, pedestrians, and, ironically, car owners is that there are too many cars. Four fifths of the world's motor vehicles are in the developed world. Saturation of markets in the West has caused a drop in the average annual rate of growth in car ownership from 5% in the 1970s to 3% in the 1980s. This still means 19 million additional cars each year, or a doubling in the number of cars every 20 years.[1] In Britain in the past 10 years the distances travelled by car and motorcycle have increased by about 40%.[5]

Many cities are now at full stretch. Average speeds are down to as low as 8 km/hour. Travelling to and from work in Mexico City can take up to four hours. According to Capital Radio's flying eye, which reports on London's traffic, the city is congested for 24 hours a day. "London is running at full capacity," said a spokesman. "It only takes a broken down lorry to cause a major snarl up." Cars also take up a lot of space. Two thirds of the land area of Los Angeles is devoted to transport in the form of roads and parking facilities.

Anything that encourages people to drive or discourages them from using alternative transport, such as bus, train, or bicycle, adds to the congestion. The high capital cost of buying, taxing, insuring, and maintaining a private car combined with the relatively low cost per kilometre encourages car owners to use their cars whenever possible. Congestion is not helped by the tendency for people to travel to work alone. Cars used for commuting contain on average 1·2-1·3 people.[6] Drivers of company cars, which tend to have bigger engines than private cars, are often relieved of all running costs. As a result company cars travel further per week than private cars.[7] These and other motoring benefits amount to a tax saving to employees of about £1·5bn a year, almost equivalent to the total government subsidy to public transport.

Motorways spawn out of town shopping and recreation facilities. Large supermarkets offer a wide selection of cheap and healthy food but are often accessible only to people with cars. Local shops cannot compete and are forced to close. Those without cars—two fifths of households in London—must either put up with a limited choice of more expensive food or invest in a car. Once bought, a car tends to be used for other journeys.

Mind the gap

Out of town shopping centres are just one example of how private cars can widen the gap between rich and poor. The benefits of travel—access to good cheap food, health and recreation facilities, and social support—are enjoyed by those doing the travelling. These tend to be people who are already socially advantaged. The health damaging effects of transport —air pollution, congestion, stress—are experienced by everyone but mostly by those in disadvantaged groups, who are more likely to live in areas of high traffic density.

Busy roads cut communities in half and block access to friends and shops, especially for young, elderly, and disabled people. Where traffic is heavy in residential streets social interactions are reduced.

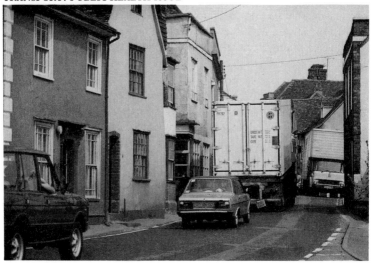

Heavy traffic reduces social interactions

The health divide is deepened not because cars protect or promote health in those who have them but because of their negative effect on those who don't.

No more roads

The growth in private car ownership also has a negative effect on other forms of transport. It makes cycling unpleasant and dangerous and reduces the use and availability of public transport. Between 1952 and 1987 the number of passenger kilometres travelled per year by car increased nearly sevenfold. Over the same period the number of passenger kilometres per year travelled by bus fell by half and that by cycle by four fifths.[2]

For this reason, the answer to traffic congestion and its attendant miseries is not simply to build more roads. This has been found to be counterproductive, most recently and dramatically with the M25 motorway round London. The initial easing of traffic flow tempts people away from public transport and into their cars. Public transport services are then used less and so go into decline forcing more people to take to their cars. Congestion builds up again, this time on a larger scale and at even slower average speeds (M J H Mogridge, lecturer at University College London, October 1985).

The real answer, as several European countries have discovered, is to discourage people as much as possible from driving cars and encourage them to use other forms of transport.

Two wheels better than four

Compared with cars, public transport is more efficient, takes up less space, uses less fuel, and produces fewer emissions. A car carrying one person needs more than seven times more energy than a bus carrying 45 people.[1] Public transport is also safer. Of all forms of road transport, buses and coaches cause fewest deaths from accidents per journey, both among the travellers and among pedestrians.[2] The quality of public transport varies widely, and this decides whether or not people use it. In Hong Kong, where public transport is cheap, reliable, and well integrated, it accounts for 9 million of the 10 million daily passenger trips.[8] In Britain between 1982 and 1988 government subsidy for road and rail transport fell by a quarter.[2]

Over two fifths of all car journeys in Britain are less than 5 km,[9] and nearly three quarters of all trips to work are less than 8 km.[10] Short trips are the most polluting as a cold engine fires inefficiently and catalytic converters only start working after about 2 km. Making these trips by bicycle or on foot would decrease air pollution and greatly reduce local traffic congestion. Journeys of 5 km are considered potentially cyclable, giving a 25 minute trip at 14 km/h—the overall speed for all cycle journeys.

In contrast with cars, bicycles do not pollute the air or create noise, they take up less space, and need no fuel other than a good breakfast.[10a] Cycling is the most energy efficient mode of transport (figure).[11] To travel 16 km a cyclist needs 1·46 MJ (350 kcal)—the amount of energy in a bowl of rice. To cover the same distance an average car needs 77·8 MJ—more than half a gallon of petrol.[12] A cyclist can ride 5·6 km on the energy found in an ear of corn. Cycling also keeps you fit. Civil servants who cycled regularly experienced half the expected number of coronary events.[13]

Cycling on a large scale already happens by necessity in the Third World. Only one in 500 Indians owns a car compared with one in two Americans. More people use bicycles in Asia than use cars in the whole world.[1] Bicycles are the perfect tool for intermediate technologists. They are cheap to produce—100 bicycles can be manufactured for the cost of one medium sized car—and can be adapted into rickshaws to carry goods or to power paddy threshers and water

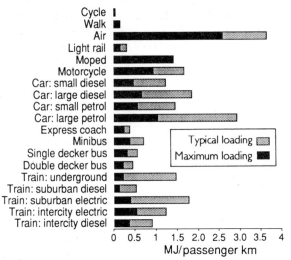

Energy consumption of various modes of transport according to maximum and normal loading[11]

pumps. China, which accounts for 300 million of the world's 800 million bicycles, has recognised the value of a self propelled workforce. People who cycle to work receive an allowance from the government. But some countries in the developing world, especially in Africa, see the bicycle as a symbol of poverty and continue to hold up the car as the ultimate form of private transport.

People in the West have bicycles but don't use them. There are seven times more bicycles in America than India but only one in 40 is used for commuting, the others are used for sport and recreation.[14] One in four people in Britain has a bicycle but only one in 33 transport trips is made by cycle.[10] There has been a fall since the 1950s, when 10% of all travel by mechanical means was by bicycle, mostly commuting to work. Now the figure is 1%, mostly for leisure.[9]

Positive action

A comparison between societies that encourage cycling and those that don't suggests that the decisions people make about transport are not related to income, technology, or degree of urban development but to enlightened public policy and strong government support.[14] Cycling is popular in the Netherlands and Denmark not just because of the weather or the flat terrain but because of positive action.

Between 1975 and 1985 the Netherlands government spent $230m building cycle routes, parking, and facilities at railways. In Dutch cities and towns 20-50% of all trips are made by bicycle. The Chinese administration provides spacious cycle lanes and easily accessible, supervised bicycle parking.

There are small signs of progress, too, from that bastion of motorists, the United States. All road repairs in the university town of Palo Alto must now comply with strict standards of smoothness, and since 1983 all new buildings over a certain size have to incorporate secure bicycle sheds and showers.

The aim should be to encourage people to make short trips by bicycle and longer trips by mass transport, with bicycles as the means of getting to and from the station. The British government has accepted proposals for 1600 km of cycle routes in London but is leaving it up to individual boroughs to implement. Meanwhile, according to Liz Marriot of the London Cycling Campaign, it is getting more not less difficult to take bicycles on trains in Britain. A flat rate of £3 per journey by Intercity is a disincentive on short journeys.

Incentives and disincentives

While most governments in the West recognise the problems of air pollution and traffic congestion, few are willing to tackle them directly by imposing restraints on private motoring. But without resorting to head on tactics there is still a wide range of measures that would act as potent disincentives to driving. The Transport and Health Study Group, a British group that campaigns for healthier transport policies, describes some of them in its policy statement.[2] Shifting the cost of motoring from capital outlay to running costs would make cars cheaper to buy but more expensive to use. More people would be able to afford cars but to use them only when absolutely necessary. This could be achieved by imposing a petrol tax instead of a licence fee, by insurance schemes related to distance travelled, or by charging for the use of roads. A carbon tax would transfer the environmental cost of motoring back on to the motorist. Withdrawing the provision of free parking at work would discourage people from commuting by car. Subsidies for company cars should also be withdrawn and companies should be encouraged to sponsor the use of public transport.

A great deal has been achieved in Germany with Verkehrsberuhigung or traffic calming measures to reduce speeds in residential areas.

Sleeping policemen and pedestrian rights of way help to enforce the impression that cars are admitted only on sufferance and that streets are for people. In Sweden, traffic is directed away from pedestrian and cycling areas.[15] The Dutch government has recently increased the cost of buying and driving a car by about half and plans to introduce an electronic system to log the number of kilometres each car travels. Excessive drivers will pay extra tax. In the longer term, town planners have a central role. Building self contained social units with houses, jobs, shopping, and recreational and health facilities within easy reach would minimise the need for travel.

The message is simple. Make it easier and more pleasant to cycle to work or use public transport and more difficult and expensive to drive. Liz Marriot does not see this approach as anti-car. Improving public transport and cycling facilities will, she thinks, benefit all road users. "At the moment if you want a car you can go out and buy one. But ultimately you can't move so it's self defeating." She acknowledges that cycling is not the answer to everyone's transport needs. "We would like to see it as part of an overall transport strategy which must include a cheap and efficient public transport system."

"Transport is a public health issue," says Judith Hanna of the Transport and Health Study Group, "just as much as clean water and clean air." We need to develop imaginative and well financed transport policies that will put the car firmly in its place as one among many options rather than the only one. Otherwise we will miss a vital opportunity to create a more equitable, humane, and healthy society.

1 Lowe M. Rethinking urban transport. In: Browne LR, ed. *State of the world 1991. A Worldwatch Institute report on progress towards a sustainable society.* London: Earthscan Publications, 1991:56-75.
2 The Public Health Alliance. *Health on the move: policies for health promoting transport. The policy statement of the Transport and Health Study Group.* Birmingham: Public Health Alliance, 1991.
3 Hillman M, Adams J, Whitelegg J. *One false move . . . a study of children's independent mobility.* London: PSI Publishing, 1990.
4 Thompson RS, Rivara FP, Thompson DC. A case-control study of the effectiveness of bicycle safety helmets. *N Engl J Med* 1989;**320**:1361-7.
5 Hillman M. Cycling and health: a policy context. In: *Cycling and the healthy city.* London: Friends of the Earth, 1990:3-13.
6 Newman P, Kenworthy J. *Cities and automobile dependence: an international sourcebook.* Aldershot: Gower, 1989.
7 Hillman M, Whalley A. *Energy and personal travel, obstacles to conservation.* London: Policy Studies Institute, 1983:185-204.
8 World Bank. *Urban transport: a World Bank policy study.* Washington, DC: World Bank, 1986.
9 Banister C. Existing travel patterns: the potential for cycling. In: *Cycling and the healthy city.* London: Friends of the Earth, 1990:20-8.

10 Clarke A. *Pro-bike: a cycling policy for the 1990s.* London: Friends of the Earth, 1987.

10a Hillman M. *Cycling: towards health and safety.* Oxford: Oxford University Press, 1992. (Report for the British Medical Association.)

11 Hughes P. Exhausting the atmosphere. *Town and Country Planning* 1991;**60**: 267-9.

12 Holcomb MC. *Transportation energy data book.* 9th ed. Oak Ridge, Tennessee: Oak Ridge National Laboratory, 1987.

13 Morris JN, Clayton DG, Everitt MG, Semmence AM, Burgess EH. Exercise in leisure time: coronary attack and death rates. *Br Heart J* 1990;**63**:325-34.

14 Lowe M. Cycling into the future. In: Browne LR, ed. *State of the world 1990. A Worldwatch Institute report on progress towards a sustainable society.* New York: W W Norton, 1990.

15 Transportation Environmental Studies. *Quality streets: how traditional urban centres benefit from traffic calming.* London: TEST, 1988.

Noise: breaking the silence

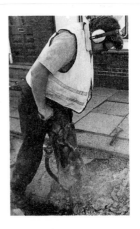

FIONA GODLEE

Last year over 100 000 complaints about noise were made to environmental health officers in England and Wales. Every year the number of complaints increases. Noise is an environmental pollutant, another product of the technological age. At high levels and over prolonged periods it damages hearing. But how dangerous is it to health?

Noise induced hearing loss

According to the United States National Institutes of Health, more than 10 million Americans have had their hearing damaged by noise, and more than 20 million are regularly exposed to levels of noise that could cause hearing loss.[1] Noise at work is the major cause of hearing loss in adults in the industrialised world.[2] In Britain the Health and Safety Executive estimates that 1·7 million people have deafness due to occupational exposure to noise. Between 1983 and 1990 almost 10 000 people in Britain qualified for disablement benefit because of noise induced hearing loss sustained at work (R H McCaig, personal communication).

A dose response relation between noise and hearing loss was established in 1970,[3] and from experimental data Professor Douglas Robinson of the Institute of Sound and Vibration Research in Southampton has estimated the risks from noise under different circumstances.[4]

It is generally accepted that noise levels below 80 dB(A) do not present a risk to hearing. A noise level of 90 dB(A), on the other hand, experienced every working day for 40 years, carries a 51% chance

Measuring noise

Noise is measured in decibels (dB). The commonly used A scale (dB(A)) incorporates a weighting to take account of the ear's varying responses to different frequencies—humans are less sensitive to low frequency sounds than to high ones. Noise is measured on a logarithmic scale. This means that a noise of 100 dB(A) has 10 times as much sound energy as one of 90 dB(A). Subjectively, an increase of 10 dB(A) makes the sound twice as loud.

The effect of background noise
With background noise at 50 dB(A) two people standing 6 m apart could engage in normal conversation. With 85 dB(A) of background noise and taking into account the fact that the voice automatically rises to compensate, a reliable face to face conversation would be possible only at a distance of less than half a metre.

of a 30 dB(A) hearing loss. Although this represents only a moderate degree of impairment, it would, says Dr Ross Coles of the Institute for Hearing Research in Nottingham, lead to considerable difficulty in following a conversation in a pub or party where there is competing background noise. At occupational noise levels of 85 dB(A) the risk of developing a 30 dB(A) loss falls to 35%. The Health and Safety Executive estimates that in Britain 2·4 million workers are exposed to levels of more than 80 dB(A).

Deafness caused by noise at work is not a twentieth century phenomenon. It was reported among metal workers more than 250 years ago and recognised in soldiers during the Napoleonic wars.[6 7] At the end of the last century it was common enough in the railway industry to be given its own name: boilermakers' deafness.[8] What is a twentieth century phenomenon, however, is the largely self inflicted damage to hearing caused by noisy social and leisure activities such as discos and personal stereos.

Disco danger

Discos are the main source of leisure noise and the most potentially damaging to hearing.[9] A report by Dr Adrian Davis and his colleagues at the Institute of Hearing Research in Nottingham estimates noise levels of about 97 dB(A) at discos, which about 6 million people attend for four hours a week for about seven years.[10] By comparison with occupational exposure the risks are small because of the shorter

75

periods of exposure. But the effects of noise on hearing are cumulative, and people who have noisy jobs tend to have noisy pastimes. In one study 10-20% of people attending discos had noisy jobs.[9] The suggestion that other factors such as tobacco and alcohol increase the risk of hearing loss from noise remains controversial.[11] Finding suitable control subjects is difficult in a society where noisy leisure pursuits tend to be associated with smoking and drinking.

Personal stereo systems are also causing concern. An estimated 5 million people use them in Britain.[10] The National Deaf Children's Society measured the maximum sound output from a selection of machines playing tapes of Mahler's *Second Symphony*.[12] All exceeded 90 dB(A) and some exceeded 100 dB(A). The headsets do not cut out background noise so when listening in noisy conditions—for example while travelling on the underground—there is a cumulative effect. This is made worse by the need to turn the volume up to compete with the background noise. In another study by Davis *et al* the sound level selected by 24 subjects was, on average, 74 dB(A) if the music was for background listening, 83 dB(A) if it was the main item of interest, and 85 dB(A) if it was rock or pop music.[10]

Davis *et al* conclude that exposure to noise during leisure activities can be equivalent to occupational exposure of 80 dB(A) over a working lifetime. For those in noisy jobs, already subjected to levels of 80 dB(A) or more, leisure noise can effectively double the risk of developing hearing loss. The Royal National Institute for the Deaf has been active in publicising the possible dangers of high output personal stereo systems, especially for young children. It is calling for warnings to be printed on the packaging of personal stereos.

After a few hours of exposure to loud noise—in a disco, for example—the ears seem to acclimatise and the noise level seems to fall. This is because noise damages the hair cells in the cochlea. Put succinctly by Professor Chris Rice, director of the Institute of Sound and Vibration Research in Southampton, "You don't become accustomed to noise, you become deaf to it."

The deafness produced by intermittent exposure to loud noise is reversible, but repeated insult can cause permanent damage. Loss of hearing due to noise begins in the high frequencies. The earliest sign is a dip in the audiometry trace at about 4000 Hz. With continued exposure the deficit spreads in both directions to higher and lower frequencies.

Damage to the hair cells in the cochlea causes tinnitus, which may precede any awareness of hearing loss. The severity of the tinnitus is

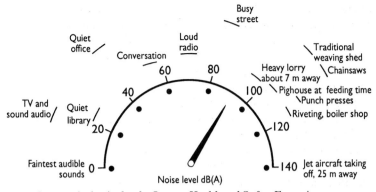

FIG 1—*Some typical noise levels. Source: Health and Safety Executive*

a good indicator of the severity of the hearing loss. Tinnitus can occur for a few minutes after exposure to loud noise—the ringing in the ears on leaving a disco, for example—or spontaneously and for longer periods. Ten per cent of adults in the United Kingdom experience spontaneous tinnitus lasting for more than five minutes.[13]

Figure 1 shows some typical noise levels. Some people seem to be more susceptible than others to the effects of noise on hearing; men are more susceptible than women, for example, although this may be a statistical quirk due to the small number of women exposed to high levels of occupational noise.[14] Brown eyed people are less susceptible than people with blue eyes, possibly because melanin on the cochlea protects it from auditory insults.[15]

Whether or not hearing loss is an inevitable consequence of aging is also controversial. Members of the primitive Mabaan tribe in Sudan are not exposed to loud noise, having no drums, let alone guns or road traffic, to contend with. Mabaan men in their 70s were found to have hearing similar to 30 year old American men who had worked in a noise free environment.[16] According to Dr Davis, however, the validity of this comparison is questionable. Professor Robinson believes that hearing loss declines naturally with age. His risk tables include one for the effects of "no noise," which predicts that one in four men in Britain will develop hearing loss of 28 dB(A) or more by the age of 60 without having been exposed to excessive noise levels.[5]

People are often reluctant to acknowledge that they are going deaf and are therefore unlikely to seek help until the problem is well advanced.[17] Problems with communication may be misinterpreted as

77

friction with other people or a change in personality. Doctors need to be aware that noise induced hearing loss is common and preventable.

Prevention

Preventing hearing loss from occupational noise is one of the jobs of the Health and Safety Executive. The 1989 Noise at Work Regulations specify two action levels above which employers have an absolute duty to reduce noise by as much as is practicable.[18] At the lower level, 85 dB(A), employers must inform employees of the dangers and explain preventive measures. Ear protectors must be provided but are worn at the employee's discretion. At levels of 90 dB(A) or more employers must ensure that ear protection is worn. Ear protectors, however, have their limitations. Their efficacy tends to be overestimated,[14] and they may interfere with communication and prevent workers from hearing warning signals.

The provision of audiometric screening in the work place is recommended but not mandatory. This, says Professor Rice, is a weakness in the law. At present employees who are worried about their hearing are advised to go to their general practitioner. As most general practitioners do not have audiometric equipment, patients are referred on to the NHS or to private audiologists. "On the principle that the polluter should pay," says Professor Rice, "this service should be provided by the employer." In making the provision of audiometry services in the workplace voluntary, the Health and Safety Executive has, he thinks, caved in under pressure from industry.

The Health and Safety Executive denies this charge. According to Dr R H McCaig, the current provision is in line with the 1986 European Community directive, which states that employees should be able to have their hearing checked by a doctor. It does not mention audiometry. The executive believes that it is better to encourage the provision of high standard audiometry on a voluntary basis than to force companies to provide it, in which case the standard may well fall.

Noise annoyance

The non-auditory effects of noise are more difficult to define. They have recently been reviewed for the Health and Safety Executive.[19] Noise annoyance consists of disturbance of normal activities such as speech and sleep. The number of complaints made by members of the public suggests that noise annoyance is on the increase (fig 2). In the past 20 years complaints about noise in Britain increased 20-fold (D Trippier, lecture to the Institution of Environmental Health Officers, September 1991). Last year local authorities in Britain received more than 100 000 serious complaints. According to a survey carried out in 1986-7 by the Building Research Establishment, noise from neighbours is the greatest source of complaints, annoying 14% of adults in England.[20] Two thirds of the noise nuisance from neighbours came from amplified music and dogs.

Reactions to environmental noise depend as much on the person as on the type and level of noise. Middle class people are more likely to be bothered by aircraft noise, for example.[21] Having some control over the level of noise, or even perceiving that you do, makes it easier to tolerate.[14]

Tolerance to noise varies enormously from person to person. A survey in London asked people whether they were annoyed by noise at home, out of doors, and at work.[22] For each setting respectively, 56%, 27%, and 20% said they were annoyed by the noise while 41%,

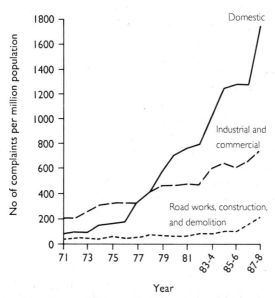

FIG 2—Noise complaints received by environmental health officers, 1971-88. Source: Environmental Health Reports, Institution of Environmental Health Officers[20]

79

64%, and 70% noticed it but were not disturbed. The rest did not even notice it. At 45 dB(A) the average opinion was "no annoyance" but 10% of people were still highly annoyed.[22]

The British 1990 Environment Protection Act has made noise a statutory nuisance like smell or smoke. Local authorities now have a statutory duty to investigate every reasonable complaint. The act also introduced draconian penalties—£2000 fine or six months in prison—for people receiving noise abatement notices and failing to act on them. Commercial companies can now be fined up to £20 000. The problem, according to a spokesman for the Noise Abatement Society, is one of enforcement. The society believes that local authorities should provide a 24 hour complaints service as most noise nuisance occurs at night.

Traffic noise

Road traffic is a major contributor to perceived environmental noise, initiating 11% of complaints to local authorities.[20] In England and Wales in 1986, the Department of the Environment recorded 11 422 offences relating to noise from motor vehicles, 90% of which involved faulty silencers.[23] Current legislation to limit noise emissions for new motor vehicles—based on a 1984 European Community directive—puts a limit of 77 dB(A) on passenger cars and 84 dB(A) on the heaviest heavy goods vehicles. Existing vehicles are simply required not to produce "excessive" noise. There is at present no provision for noise checks as part of the Department of Transport test (MOT), although, according to Mr Andrew Brown of the department's vehicle standards and engineering division, this is being considered.

As with air pollution, tightening up on noise emissions from individual vehicles will have little effect on overall noise levels if the volume of traffic continues to grow. The United States Environmental Protection Agency is recommending that overall outdoor noise should be limited to an average of 55 dB(A) to prevent noise annoyance.[14]

Sleep disturbance

Interference with sleep is the commonest form of annoyance caused by noise. But measuring its extent and effects is fraught with difficulty. The artificial surroundings of the sleep laboratory inevitably alter subjects' reactions, while responses to questionnaires about noise and sleep tend to be highly subjective. Added to this is the

80

problem that not all sleep disturbance is due to noise. According to a survey in Greater London, 20% of people suffer from sleep disturbance unrelated to noise.[24]

The type and timing of the noise is important. Intermittent noises or changes in noise level—as happens when an aeroplane passes overhead—are more disturbing than continuous noise of an equivalent energy level; and meaningful sounds, such as the cry of a child, are more likely to disturb sleep than neutral sounds. Sensitivity to sleep disruption due to noise is about 10 dB(A) lower in children than in adults, which means that children suffer less. The early hours of the morning are the worst time, especially for elderly people, because this is the time of lightest sleep.[14]

Sleep disturbance can mean that the person takes longer to fall asleep, wakes repeatedly, or is aware of having slept badly the next morning. Peak noise levels of 60 dB(A)—for example, from passing traffic—or an ambient level of 50 dB(A) may greatly increase the time taken to fall asleep.[25] Noise may also cause changes of which the person is unaware, such as shifts from heavy to lighter sleep, reductions in rapid eye movement sleep, and increases in body movements during the night.[14 26]

The effects of a bad night's sleep include mood change, reduced cardiovascular performance, and poor performance at intellectual and mechanical tasks. A recent review of research into noise and sleep recommends that sound at night in sleeping quarters should not exceed 45 dB(A).[14]

Noise can have positive effects. It increases arousal and may improve concentration and performance of simple, repetitive tasks, especially when the person is sleepy or unmotivated.[27] But noise worsens performance of complex or intellectual tasks. Fewer accidents occur when noise levels are reduced[27]; and American schoolchildren whose classrooms looked out on to railway lines performed less well in reading tests than similar children in classrooms on the quiet side of the school.[14] Noise also adversely affects behaviour, increasing anxiety and reducing the incidence of helpful behaviour.[14] Levels of aggression are increased by loud noise, an effect which may persist outside the noisy environment. Steelworkers have more domestic disputes if they work in noisy areas.[14]

Noise and psychiatric problems

Studies have shown a consistent relation between sensitivity to noise and psychiatric illness.[28] But there is no evidence that noise actually causes psychiatric problems. High scores on the general health questionnaire—indicating psychiatric illness—were associated with degree of annoyance due to noise rather than with the degree of noise itself.[29] Dr Stephen Stansfield and his colleagues at the Institute of Psychiatry in London found that women who were highly sensitive to noise had significantly more psychiatric symptoms, higher scores for neuroticism, and greater reactivity to other stimuli such as air pollution than women who were less sensitive to noise.[30] In a study of people suffering from depression, sensitivity to noise fell when patients recovered.[31] Stansfield concludes that sensitivity to noise acts as a non-specific marker for increased vulnerability to other stresses in the environment.

Other effects of noise

The idea that noise might jeopardise physical health became the subject of controversy in the 1980s with the publication of data suggesting increased mortality related to noise near Los Angeles International Airport. Subsequent reports found the analysis to be faulty,[32] but other studies claim to have found links between noise and several diseases including stroke, cardiovascular disease, hypertension, and peptic ulceration.[33] Experimental studies have also shown that noise can produce changes in circulation and skin resistance.[34]

There are good theoretical reasons why noise might cause such effects. It triggers the so called fight or flight mechanisms in the body, causing cardiovascular and other autonomic changes. The relation between stress and illness is now well recognised, and stress is known to be exacerbated by feelings of lack of control, such as those caused by noise inflicted by others. But assessing whether a widespread and varied environmental factor like noise contributes to common diseases is difficult. There are problems with potential confounders—smoking, alcohol, diet, age, pre-existing illness, other environmental factors—and with finding unexposed control subjects. In addition, extrapolations from experimental data, whether on humans or animals, are not always valid. In a critical review of all published studies that examined the effects of noise on cardiovascular health, Shirley Thompson of the University of South Carolina concluded that the only consistent finding was a small increase in blood pressure.[35]

Interpreting the findings creates further controversy. What, for example, might be the long term implications of a temporary increase in blood pressure due to noise? This question is now being addressed by the Medical Research Council's Caerphilly and Speedwell Prospective Heart Disease Studies.[36] So far, according to Dr Peter Ellwood, director of the council's epidemiology unit in South Glamorgan, the findings relating to noise are inconclusive.

Conclusion

Noise damages hearing. Environmental noise probably contributes little to the overall risk of hearing loss, except where loud music is concerned. Low levels of noise in the environment can, however, damage health in the wider sense of wellbeing. Noise also contributes to the dehumanising effect of our increasingly urban society.

1 National Institutes of Health. *Noise and hearing loss. Consensus statement.* Vol 8. Washington, DC: NIH, 1990:1-24.

2 Phaneuf R, Hetu R. An epidemiological perspective of the causes of hearing loss among industrial workers. *J Otolaryngol* 1990;**19**:31-40.

3 Burns W, Robinson DW. *Hearing and noise in industry.* London: HMSO, 1970.

4 Robinson DW. *Noise exposure and hearing: a new look at the experimental data.* London: HMSO, 1987.

5 Robinson DW. *Tables for the estimation of hearing impairment due to noise for otologically normal persons and for a typical unscreened population as a function of age and duration of exposure.* London: HMSO, 1988.

6 Ramazzini B. *Diseases of workers.* New York: Hafner, 1968. *De morbus artificum.* (Translated by W C Wright.)

7 Fosbroke J. Practical observations on the pathology and treatment of deafness. *Lancet* 1831;i:645-8.

8 Atherley G, Noble W. Occupational deafness: the continuing challenge of early German and Scottish research. *Am J Ind Med* 1985;**8**:101-7.

9 Bickerdike J, Gregory A. *An evaluation of hearing damage risk to attenders at discotheques.* Leeds: School of Constructional Studies, Leeds Polytechnic, 1979.

10 Davis AC, Fortnum HM, Coles RRA, Hagard MP, Lutman ME. *Damage to hearing arising from leisure noise: a review of the literature.* London: HMSO, 1985.

11 Barone JA, Peters JM, Garabrant DH, Burnstein L, Crebsbach R. Smoking as a risk factor in noise induced hearing loss. *J Occup Med* 1987;**29**:741-5.

12 National Deaf Children's Society. *Personal stereos and children's hearing.* London: NDCS, 1990.

13 Davis AC. The prevalence of hearing impairment and reported hearing disability among adults in Great Britain. *Int J Epidemiol* 1989;**18**:911-7.

14 Suter AH. Noise and its effects. In: Shapiro SA. *The Dormant Noise Control Act and options to abate noise pollution.* Washington, DC: Administrative Conference of the United States, 1991.

15 Carter NL. Eye colour and susceptibility to noise induced permanent threshold shift. *Audiology* 1980;**19**:86-93.

16 Beales PH. *Noise, hearing and deafness.* London: Michael Joseph, 1965.

17 Hetu R, Getty L. Coping with occupational hearing loss: the University of Montreal acoustics groups rehabilitation programme. In: *Occupational noise induced hearing loss: prevention and rehabilitation.* Sydney: National Occupational Health and Safety Commission, 1991.

18 Health and Safety Executive. *Noise at Work Regulations 1989*. London: HMSO, 1990.

19 Smith A. *Non auditory effects of noise at work: a review of the literature*. London: Health and Safety Executive, 1991. (HSE contract research 30.)

20 Department of the Environment. *Report of the Noise Review Working Party 1990*. London: HMSO, 1990.

21 Office of Population Censuses and Surveys, Social Survey Division. *Second survey of aircraft noise annoyance around London (Heathrow) Airport*. London: HMSO, 1979.

22 Large JB. Methods of assessing community response to environmental noise. *R Soc Health J* 1977;**97**:147-52.

23 Department of the Environment. *Digest of environmental protection and water statistics 1987*. London: HMSO, 1988.

24 Langdon FJ, Buller IB. Road traffic noise and disturbance to sleep. *J Sound Vibration* 1977;**50**:13-28.

25 Vernet M. Effect of train noise on sleep for people living in homes bordering the railway line. *J Sound Vibration* 1979;**66**:483-92.

26 Vallet M. Psychophysiological effects of exposure to aircraft or road traffic noise. *Proceedings of the Institute of Acoustics* 1979;**3**:1-4.

27 Broadbent D. Human performance in noise. In: Harris C, ed. *Handbook of noise control*. 2nd ed. New York: McGraw-Hill, 1978:1-19.

28 Tarnopolsky A, Barker SM, Wiggins RO, McLean EK. The effect of aircraft noise on the mental health of a community. *Psychol Med* 1978;**8**:219-33.

29 Tarnopolsky A, Morton-Williams J. *Aircraft noise and prevalence of psychiatric disorders*. London: Social and Community Planning Research, 1980.

30 Stansfield SA, Clarke CR, Jenkins LM, Tarnopolsky A. Sensitivity to noise in a community sample: measurement of psychiatric disorder and personality. *Psychol Med* 1985;**15**:243-54.

31 Stansfield SA. Noise sensitivity, depressive illness, and personality: a longitudinal study in depressed patients with matching control subjects. In: Burgland B, ed. *Proceedings of the fifth international congress on noise as a public health problem*. Vol 3. Stockholm: Karolinska Institute, 1988:339-44.

32 Frerichs RR, Beeman BL, Coulson AH. Los Angeles airport noise and mortality — faulty analysis and public policy. *Am J Public Health* 1980;**70**: 357-62.

33 United Nations Environmental Programme and World Health Organisation. *Environmental health criteria 12. Noise*. Geneva: WHO, 1980.

34 Bastnier H, Klosterkoetter W, Large JB. *Environment and the quality of life. Damage and annoyance caused by noise*. Brussels: Commission of the European Communities, 1975. (EUR 5398e.)

35 Thompson SJ. Effects of noise on the cardiovascular system: appraisal of epidemiological evidence. In: Rossi G, ed. *Noise as a public health problem. Proceedings of the fourth international congress*. Vol 1. Milan: Centra Richerche e Studi Amplifon, 1983:711-4.

36 Medical Research Council Epidemiology Unit. *Epidemiological studies of cardiovascular diseases: Progress report VII 1991*. MRC: Cardiff, 1991.

Drinking water: doubts about quality

ALISON WALKER

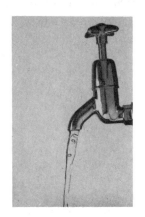

Does anyone trust tap water any more? Sales of bottled mineral water increased from three million to 128 million litres between 1976 and 1986, and a survey of over 250 people in London and the midlands in 1988 showed that over a quarter never drank water direct from the tap.[1] The water industry, feeling the consequences of privatisation, stringent European Community directives, and growing pressure from environmental groups, is finding it hard to convince the public that tap water is still safe, let alone palatable. Scares like the accidental contamination of water at Camelford with aluminium have not helped either. But are the public's fears justified? Is drinking water any less safe than it was 50 years ago?

Water sources

Some impurities in tap water are inevitable. These derive both from the different sources of water and from the treatment process.

Domestic water is extracted from groundwater, reservoirs, or rivers depending on local geography.[2] Groundwater is pumped up from aquifers or water permeable rocks. These are mostly found in the chalk regions of the south of England and the sandstones of the east midlands. They provide nearly a third of the water in England and Wales. Natural filtering takes place through the rock, but contamination is still possible. Supplies from aquifers near waste disposal sites, for example, may be contaminated if drainage water from the

85

sites percolates through them. A survey carried out by the Department of the Environment in 1987 of 100 landfill sites in Britain showed that a disturbingly high percentage (62%) took no measures to prevent groundwater ingress.[3] Groundwater in agricultural areas is also at increased risk of contamination because nitrate based fertilisers and pesticides can leach into the supply.

Reservoirs are mainly found in upland areas of Scotland, Wales, northern England, and the south west, where the local geography makes damming of valleys practicable. The water tends to be soft and peaty and is relatively uncontaminated, being situated away from industrial areas.

Rivers such as the Thames, Ouse, and Severn provide water for the dense urban populations of the towns and cities located nearby. River water is often recycled through sewage works and used again by towns further downstream (box). Britain is fortunate in being an island—the river pollution problems faced in this country are dwarfed by those in countries bordering on international rivers such as the Rhine in Europe.

Water treatment

No set procedure exists for water treatment as water varies so much around the country, but in general groundwater needs less treatment than surface water. A preliminary storage stage (during which most bacteria will die) may begin the treatment but is not incorporated into all plants. Modern plants of various designs are based on chemical coagulation—for example, with aluminium sulphate—followed by sedimentation and filtration. Other stages are added to remove iron

---

River pollution in Britain

Class 1a—High quality suitable for potable supply and all other abstractions; game and other high class fisheries; high amenity value.
Class 1b—Less high quality than class 1a but usable for substantially the same purposes.
Class 2—Suitable for potable supply after advanced treatment; supporting reasonably good coarse fisheries; moderate amenity value.
Class 3—Polluted to an extent that fish are absent or only sporadically present; may be used for low grade industrial abstraction; considerable potential for further use if cleaned up.
Class 4—Grossly polluted and likely to cause a nuisance.

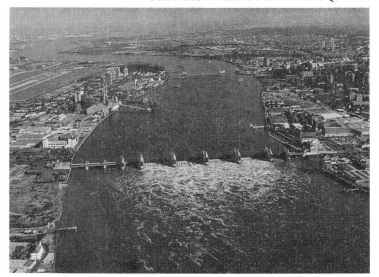

How many times will this water have been recycled before it reaches the sea?

and manganese, to control taste and odour, and to remove organic matter. Older treatment plants use slow sand filtration through several layers of finely graded sand, but because these require substantial areas of land and have high labour costs no new plants of this type have been installed for years. The final stage in all treatment works is disinfection. Chlorine is the commonest disinfectant used, although ozone or exposure to ultraviolet light are becoming more popular. Before water leaves the treatment works its pH and hardness are adjusted and fluoride may also be added.

Serious accidental contamination of drinking water either before or at the treatment works is fortunately rare. Much more of a public health concern are the possible long term effects of long term exposure to substances present in drinking water at low concentrations. Legislation exists to regulate the concentration of these impurities, and the task of adhering to required standards falls to the water industry.

The water industry

The water industry in Britain was privatised in 1989. Drinking water is now supplied by 10 regional water service companies and 29 smaller water companies, all of which have a statutory duty to provide wholesome water to the public.[5] Though the water industry

87

has always been a target for environmental campaigners, pressure on it has increased since privatisation. The water companies are required to comply with physical, chemical, and biological standards for water intended for drinking, washing, and cooking purposes as defined by the European Community drinking water directive. Sixty six variables are described in the directive of mandatory standards for all European suppliers (box). While the water companies seek derogations or exemptions from some of the standards they consider to be too stringent, pressure groups and the media are quick to point to companies finding difficulties with compliance—and are able to feed the public's anxieties.

The Department of the Environment has issued a programme for improving drinking water, which is intended to bring virtually all drinking water supplies up to standard by 1995. A total of £1·8bn is being invested over the next five years—which ultimately will have to be paid by the customer. In the meantime water companies can apply for derogations in circumstances where the nature of the source from which the water is extracted makes it difficult to comply with the European Community directive or where there is a delay while steps are taken to ensure compliance with microbiological and toxic levels.

One of the toughest standards is for pesticides. Maximum admissible concentrations of pesticides in water of 0·1 μg/l for individual pesticides and 0·5 μg/l for the total pesticide concentration are required by the European Community directive. In 1990, 34 pesticides were detected at concentrations above 0·1 μg/l by the government's drinking water inspectorate.[6] The pesticides most often detected are those used on roadside verges and railways, such as atrazine and simazine. The low levels required by the directive amount to a virtual ban on pesticides in water, according to Peter Matthews, director of quality at Anglian Water. Professor Ronald Packham, former chief scientist at the Water Research Centre,

---

Key variables used for the assessment of water quality

Coliforms	Odour	Aluminium	Polycyclic aromatic
Faecal coliforms	(quantitative)	Iron	hydrocarbons
Colour	Taste	Manganese	(PAH)
Turbidity	(quantitative)	Lead	Pesticides
	Nitrate		

believes that the directive is inflexible and suffers from having no built in scheme for revision. World Health Organisation guidelines laid down in 1984, he says, were far more realistic and even then had an enormous safety factor. The media, he added, have tended to highlight instances of non-compliance, equating them with a health hazard—which is not necessarily the case.

Health risks

While disputes continue over legislation governing drinking water standards, medical evidence linking contamination with possible health risks has been gathering, although it is still limited.

Little doubt exists over the health risk from the presence of some contaminants in drinking water; infectious diseases, for example, are known to be transmitted by a wide range of microorganisms found in contaminated water. For chemical constituents the picture is not always clear. Some chemicals can now be detected in drinking water at concentrations of a million billionth of a gram per litre. In many cases, however, the ability to detect these substances in water has outstripped our knowledge of their medical significance.

Microbiological contaminants

John Snow elegantly showed the waterborne cause of the 1854 cholera epidemic in London by removing the handle of the Broad Street water pump. Any microorganism transmitted by the faecal-oral route has the potential to cause infection, but modern water treatment plants aim at disinfecting water sufficiently before it reaches the public. *Escherichia coli* is tested for as an indicator of possible faecal contamination before water leaves the treatment plant.

A review of outbreaks of waterborne disease in Sweden from 1975 to 1984 showed that in almost all cases the causes were technical hitches at the treatment plants.[7] These included broken sewage pipes, blockage of wastewater pipes, or sudden pollution of water intakes coinciding with inadequate chlorination. Although campylobacter was the most commonly identified causative organism, previously ignored pathogens such as giardia, Norwalk agents, and cryptosporidium have been shown to be important in the past few years.

Cryptosporidium has also been incriminated as the cause of contaminated drinking water in Britain. In 1989 an outbreak of cryptosporidiosis in Swindon and Oxford "caught the water industry napping," according to some critics. The organism is thought to have entered the water supply after the Thames was contaminated with farmyard slurry. Most people exposed to the parasite simply develop a self limiting gastroenteritis lasting up to a week, but in immuno-compromised patients it can cause severe diarrhoea and dehydration. The organism survives chlorine treatment and is not routinely tested for at treatment plants. Tap water was incriminated as the cause of the outbreak in the Thames region, naturally causing public concern. The incident was fully investigated by an expert panel chaired by Sir John Badenoch.[8]

Bottled waters have also come under scrutiny.[8a] Micro-organisms have been isolated in them, although only those that are non-pathogenic under normal conditions. Lower total viable counts of organisms are found in carbonated waters because of the known antibacterial activity of carbon dioxide in water.

Chemical contaminants

The risks of chemical contamination of drinking water are not as clearly understood as those of microbiological contamination. Nevertheless environmental pressure groups will argue that pioneers in public health campaigned for cleaner water long before the pathogens causing infectious disease were discovered. Already some chemicals in water supplies are known to be potentially harmful.[9]

Aluminium

Many water treatment works add aluminium sulphate to the water as a coagulant to help remove suspended matter. Most of the aluminium is removed in the subsequent filtration and clarification processes, but residual amounts may pass into the water supply. The current European Community directive specifies a maximum acceptable concentration of 0·2 mg/l, although this level is based on the incidence of dirty water problems and not on health effects.

Most evidence surrounding the health risks from aluminium in drinking water link it with neurotoxicity and particularly Alzheimer's disease. "Dialysis dementia" has been described in patients on renal dialysis using water with a high concentration of aluminium. More recent epidemiological evidence showed that the risk of Alzheimer's disease was 1·5 times higher in districts where the mean aluminium concentration in drinking water was greater than 0·11 mg/l compared with districts where it was less than 0·01 mg/l.[10] This study has been criticised for several reasons, including for ignoring family history, for having a low case ascertainment, for ignoring patients who had not had computed tomography, and for being too simplistic.

Only a few people consumed large amounts of water after the accident at the Lowermoor works in Camelford in 1988 when a lorry driver mistakenly discharged 20 tonnes of concentrated aluminium sulphate solution into the wrong tank. Up to 400 people still complain of symptoms, but whether this accident helps to clarify anything other than the acute effects of aluminium poisoning remains debatable.[11]

Nitrate

The maximum admissible concentration for nitrate in drinking water is 50 mg/l and is based on the risk of bottle fed infants developing methaemoglobinaemia. Nitrate in water can be converted in the stomach to nitrite, which readily combines with fetal haemoglobin converting it to methaemoglobin. When 10% of the total haemoglobin is in the methaemoglobin form, cyanosis occurs. Levels above 70% are lethal. Methaemoglobinaemia is extremely rare and there have been no cases of high nitrate causing any deaths in Britain since 1948.[12]

A more contentious issue is the link between gastric cancer and nitrate in the diet. Vegetables and drinking water are two of the main dietary sources of nitrate and nitrite, the other major source being the preservatives added to meat to prevent botulism and to enhance colour. Nitrate can be converted to nitrite by bacteria in the mouth and stomach. This nitrite in turn can be converted to N-nitroso compounds, most of which are strongly carcinogenic in animals. International comparisons relate high levels of nitrate exposure to mortality from gastric cancer — for example, in Denmark, Hungary, and Italy. The findings have not always been consistent, and in Britain studies have not confirmed that environmental nitrates and nitrites play a major part in the risk of gastric cancer.[13] The discovery that nitrate is synthesised in humans and that nitric oxide is a natural endogenous mediator of cellular communications[14] raises further questions over the significance of exogenous nitrate in cancer.

Lead

Most houses built before 1964 have some lead pipework. People most at risk from contaminated water supplies are those living in older houses in areas with acidic water, which include Scotland, the north of England, Wales, and the west country.[12] There is little doubt about the toxicity of lead. The effects of short term, high dose exposure are well established, causing among other things abdominal pain, headache, irritability, and eventually coma and death. But the effect of long term low exposure is not fully known.

The main concern is over the possible relation between exposure to lead and behavioural and learning difficulties in children. Since the first studies in the late 1970s evidence has accumulated pointing to an inverse relation between blood lead concentrations and measures of intelligence.[15] A general lowering of the acceptable concentration for lead in drinking water is likely to occur in the future.

Hardness of water

Calcium, nitrate, silica, and conductivity are among the variables which correlate strongly with water hardness. Epidemiological evidence has shown an inverse relation between the hardness of water and mortality from cardiovascular disease—towns with very soft water were shown to have about 10% higher mortality than towns with harder water after taking into account age, sex, and socio-economic and climatic factors.[16] Houses fitted with water softeners should keep one tap supplying hard water for cooking and drinking.

Pesticides

In 1990, amid much publicity, the BMA reported on the possible health risks of pesticides.[12] Having comprehensively reviewed the literature, the association found that most studies of the long term effects of pesticides were inconclusive and that more specific information was needed. The BMA report prompted a new green card reporting system with a central Pesticides Incident Monitoring Unit. The green card is analogous to the yellow card system already used to gather information about adverse drug reactions. Using the green card system, doctors should report evidence of adverse effects from exposure to pesticides in their patients to the new monitoring unit. This replaces previous arrangements whereby several agencies collected data in an uncoordinated way. The new unit will be able to monitor the effects of exposure to pesticides on the public and improve the current level of knowledge on the toxicity of pesticides.

Conclusion

The media, fuelled by environmental pressure groups, urge the government to ensure that water resources are not polluted, that water treatment works do not save money by cutting corners, and that water quality comes up to standard. On the other hand the water industry continues to try to reassure the public that drinking water remains as good as it was 50 years ago, if not better. The results of two recent surveys have lent support to the industry, finding tap water to be mostly of good quality although with a few exceptions. One report from the Drinking Water Inspectorate found that standards were met in 99% of the 3·3 million tests it carried out in England and Wales in 1990. It also, however, was considering prosecuting four water companies for failure to meet drinking water standards. Another survey of London's drinking water in 1989 by the Institution of Environmental Health Officers found that nearly 60% of the samples taken failed to comply with the standard for the herbicides atrazine and simazine.[17] Yet the report was still able to conclude that, overall, London's water was "wholesome" with no risk to health.

The decision whether to trust tap water is ultimately left up to the consumer. But if fad or simply fancy advertising persuades you to buy bottled water, spare a thought for your purse. A litre of bottled water may cost 50p or more, while a litre of tap water costs as little as 0·03p.

1 Wheeler D. Risk assessment and the public perception of water quality. *Annual symposium of the Institution of Water and Environmental Management*. London: IWEM, 1990:2-1—2-13.

2 Hall C. *Running water*. London: Robertson McCarta, 1989.

3 Croft B, Campbell D. Characteristics of 100 landfill sites. In: *Proceedings of 1990 Harwell waste management symposium*. Harwell: United Kingdom Atomic Energy Authority, 1990.

5 Water Services Association. *Waterfacts*. London: Water Services Association, 1990.

6 Department of the Environment. *Drinking water 1990 — a report by the chief inspector, drinking water inspectorate*. London: HMSO, 1991.

7 Andersson Y, Stenströ TA. Waterborne outbreaks in Sweden—causes and etiology. *Water Science and Technology* 1987;**19**:575-80.

8 Group of Experts. *Report on cryptosporidium in water supplies*. London: HMSO, 1990.

8a Richards J, Stokely D, Hipgrave P. Quality of drinking water. *BMJ* 1992;**304**:571.

9 Packham RF. Chemical aspects of water quality and health. *Annual symposium of the Institution of Water and Environmental Management*. London: IWEM, 1990:4-1—4-15.

10 Martyn C, Osmond C, Edwardson JA. Geographical relation between Alzheimer's disease and aluminium in drinking water. *Lancet* 1989;i:59-62.

11 Lowermoor Health Advisory Group. *Water pollution at Lowermoor North Cornwall. Second report*. London: HMSO, 1990.

12 British Medical Association. *Pesticides, chemicals, and health*. London: Edward Arnold, 1990.

13 Forman D, Al-Dabbagh S, Doll R. Nitrates, nitrites and gastric cancer in Great Britain. *Nature* 1985;**313**:620-5.

14 Collier J, Vallance P. Physiological importance of nitric oxide. *BMJ* 1991;**302**: 1289-90.
15 Lee WR, Moore MR. Low level exposure to lead. *BMJ* 1990;**301**:504-5.
16 Pocock SJ, Shaper AG, Cook DG, Packham RF, Lacey RI, Powell P, *et al*. British Regional Heart Study: geographic variations in cardiovascular mortality, and the role of water quality. *BMJ* 1980;**280**:1243-8.
17 Working party on London wide drinking water. *London's drinking water*. London: Institution of Environmental Health Officers, 1990.

Swimming: hazards of taking a dip

ALISON WALKER

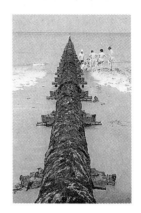

> In summer it [the sewage] causes a visible brown buoyant stain extending from the outfall pipe and spreading its way along the bays as it is brought in by the incoming tide.
>
> Sons of Neptune bathing club, Scarborough[1]

Scarborough is not the only resort where holidaymakers have to contend with sewage in the sea. Short Victorian outfall pipes still discharge sewage from coastal towns all round Britain. Leaving Britain's shores and holidaying in the Mediterranean provides no escape as the beaches there are no better. The picture, however, is changing. The long held belief that the sea can absorb, dilute, and disperse everything discharged into it is now seen as wishful thinking and is no longer accepted. Throughout Europe resorts are starting to be cleaned up as European politicians begin to take notice of public opinion and growing scientific evidence incriminating contaminated sea water as the cause of symptoms in holidaymakers.

Health risks from swimming in seawater

Until a few years ago the British government relied on research from the 1950s to form the cornerstone of its policy on bathing water. The research was performed by the Public Health Laboratory Service and looked retrospectively at poliomyelitis (a serious problem at that time) and enteric fever in sea bathers. The conclusions were reported jointly by the laboratory service and the Medical Research Council and showed that, with the exception of a few heavily polluted waters, the risk to public health from swimming in sea water contaminated by sewage could, for all practical purposes, be ignored.[2]

Things have moved on since the 1950s, and although the laboratory service's studies were carefully conducted, they are now seen to be limited by the techniques of the time. The risk of swimming in heavily polluted water remains undisputed and carries with it the risk of contracting infections such as typhoid, shigellosis, leptospirosis, and hepatitis A. More contentious, however, is the possible link between minor infections and swimming in sea water that is only moderately contaminated.

Establishing a link between minor illnesses such as gastroenteritis and ear, nose, and throat infections and swimming in polluted sea water is extremely difficult because these conditions are so common and may have various causes. Some headway has been made from large epidemiological studies which have compared the symptoms of swimmers with those of people who stayed out of the water.

One of the first studies to show a relation between sea bathing and minor symptoms was a prospective cohort study carried out in the 1970s by the United States Environmental Protection Agency.[3] The work was performed by Victor Cabelli in three different resorts — New York City, Lake Pontchartrain, Louisiana, and Boston — over five years. Altogether more than 25 000 people took part. Those bathing were questioned about symptoms acquired after swimming in the sea, and members of their family and friends who did not swim were used as controls. Samples of seawater were also taken and tested for levels of contamination. Cabelli's results showed a relation between swimming, gastrointestinal symptoms, and the quality of the sea water. This study, like most later studies, had to use self reporting of symptoms without any medical check ups or clinical tests to confirm these symptoms. In a pilot study Cabelli had found that volunteers could not be persuaded to submit to a free medical examination.

Cabelli's work spawned other studies around the world from researchers attempting to obtain repeatable and reliable quantifiable data. Although repeated with only varying degrees of success, Cabelli's method of using a prospective cohort study with self reported symptoms has since been endorsed by the World Health Organisation and United Nations environmental programme.

British studies

In Britain the Department of the Environment, cofunded by the

National Rivers Authority and the Welsh Office, commissioned its own research in 1989 to assess the risks associated with swimming in polluted sea water. Two types of study were performed—a beach study similar to that used by Cabelli (but with better statistical analysis) and their own healthy volunteer cohort study, which included medical check ups and clinical tests to confirm the results of reported symptoms. The work was headed by Dr Edmond Pike, principal microbiologist at the Water Research Centre, in conjunction with the Robens Institute at the University of Surrey and St David's University College, Lampeter.

Pilot studies were first carried out at Langland Bay in West Glamorgan to assess the two methods.[4] In the beach survey more than 4000 people on the beach during 20 days in August were interviewed about perceived symptoms and bathing histories. A week later nearly 800 of them were telephoned to obtain further information about any symptoms. Intensive microbiological sampling of the water was carried out on the days of the beach survey. The second method, the cohort study, recruited just over 270 people. They first underwent clinical tests before bathing (throat, ear, and nose swabs and faecal samples were taken) and then were interviewed for symptoms of ill health on the day they went swimming. Finally, the interviews and clinical tests were repeated three days after exposure. A further postal interview and faecal sample were obtained four weeks after exposure.

Results from both phases of the study at Langland Bay showed a higher incidence of ear and throat symptoms among those who went into the sea. The studies were not designed to produce statistically valid results but to confirm the effectiveness of the methods. Nevertheless, some significant results did emerge. The beach survey, for example, found that 1 in 13 bathers reported symptoms compared with only 1 in 32 non-bathers. Furthermore, the study indicated that the rate of reporting one or more symptoms was related to the degree of contact with the water. The results of the cohort survey did not show any correlation between reported symptoms and the results of the medical check up or analysis of the throat, ear, and nose swabs and faecal samples taken. This part of the study, however, said Dr Pike, was hampered by having a big drop out rate between volunteering and the day of exposure.

The Department of the Environment's report of the Langland Bay studies was presented to the House of Commons Environment Committee in 1990. The committee had been given the task of investigating the pollution of Britain's beaches.[1] In its conclusion it was critical of the lack of interest shown by past governments, saying that Britain's reputation abroad had been damaged. It went on to recommend that the Water Research Centre carry out further larger studies in order to be able to quantify the level of risk to bathers. These were performed in 1990 at Ramsgate Sands in Kent, where a beach survey was carried out, and Moreton Beach in Merseyside, where a healthy volunteer cohort study was performed. These studies formed the first stage of a definitive study to establish a relation between microbiological quality of sea water and the risks to health of bathers.

Both the Ramsgate Sands and the Moreton Beach studies yielded significant conclusions despite their small sample sizes.[5] At both Moreton and Ramsgate bathers were more likely to suffer from minor infections than non-bathers, and a dose related risk was established — waders experiencing fewer symptoms than swimmers, who in turn were less ill than surfers and divers. The success of these studies has led to extension of the work to include eight beaches in 1991 and 1992 and interviews with over 16 000 holiday makers.[6]

One of the main findings of the study at Ramsgate was the significant association between bathing in the sea and gastrointestinal symptoms.[7] The sea water at Ramsgate contains a high level of faecal pollution and, of some political concern, has failed the European Commission bathing water directive standards for two years running.

European Commission bathing water directive

The European Commission bathing water directive was introduced in 1975. It defines standards for beaches authorised for bathing or where bathing is "not prohibited and is traditionally practised by large numbers of bathers." All European Community members had 10 years in which to bring their beaches up to scratch. Only 27 beaches were initially identified by the British government as affected by the directive, which, unrealistically, ignored resorts like Brighton and Blackpool. In 1987, more than 10 years later, the government conceded and a further 350 beaches were included. In 1991, 453 beaches were identified as bathing waters in Britain. No bathing waters have been designated inland (box).

The directive defines physical, chemical, and microbiological standards for bathing water based on the results of fortnightly samples taken during the bathing seasons from April to September. The tests are carried out in Britain by the National Rivers Authority, reporting

Swimming inland

No inland waters are designated for bathing. The only regular monitoring that takes place in them is of chemical and not microbiological variables. Although there were no statutory requirements for the National Rivers Authority to test inland waters, monitoring does take place in some non-designated inland waters used for recreational purposes.[8] In general, river waters do not meet the coliform criteria of the European Commission bathing water directive because of the presence of treated sewage effluents and other agricultural inputs. Many of the inland still waters and abandoned docks, however, are of high bacteriological quality.

An old problem has recently re-emerged in rivers, estuaries, and the sea—that of toxins released by blooms of certain cyanobacteria (blue green algae). The death of some dogs in 1989 who drank contaminated water from Rutland reservoir, brought the subject back on to the front page. An increased nutrient load of phosphates and nitrates from sewage works, together with the long hot summers of recent years, is believed to have promoted the excessive growth of cyanobacteria. For the past two years the rivers authority has been monitoring waters for algae. Of the 680 tested, nearly 600 were found to contain cyanobacteria but only 170 of them contained high densities of bacteria. Furthermore, not all cyanobacteria release toxins—and predicting whether a particular bloom will be toxic or not is impossible.[9] Those that are produce three types of toxin—neurotoxins, hepatotoxins, and contact irritants. That they can be lethal has been shown by the death of animals, but more research is needed before the risks can be better understood. At present the best approach is prevention, as emphasised in the authority's report on toxic cyanobacteria,[10] and avoidance of water containing algal scum.

to the Department of the Environment.[8] Table I summarises the microbiological standards.[11] The recent results have shown that 76% of Britain's beaches complied with the directive in 1991 compared with 77% in 1990. The figure for 1990 was below the figure for other European countries in that year, notably the Netherlands (90%), France (86%), and Ireland (85%).[12] Nevertheless, the government has set in motion an improvement programme costing £2bn to make sure that virtually all bathing waters will be up to standard by the end of 1995. This has necessitated a review by undertakers of sewage treatment before discharge into the sea.

Sewage treatment

Up until 1990 most sewage from coastal areas in Britain was

TABLE 1—*Microbiological standards of European Community bathing water directive (95% of samples should contain these levels[11])*

	Guide level	Mandatory level	Minimum sampling frequency
Total coliforms/100 ml	500	10 000	Fortnightly
Faecal coliforms/100 ml	100	2000	Fortnightly
Faecal streptococci/100 ml	100		Discretionary
Salmonella/l		0	Discretionary
Enteroviruses (plaque forming units/10l)		0	Discretionary

discharged straight into the sea with the only treatment, if any, being that of screening for the removal of gross solids, or maceration.[8] Short and long sea outfall pipes and stormwater overflows are the three main routes by which sewage is discharged direct into the sea. In March 1990 it was announced that a minimum of primary treatment (box) would be required before sewage effluent was discharged into the sea. This has now been introduced as another European Commission directive, the municipal waste water directive, which was passed in April 1991 and now applies to all member states.

Even once the new directive has been fully implemented and sewage effluent is treated before being discharged into the sea, the possibility of some contamination of seawater remains. Primary sewage treatment will remove only 30-80% of pathogens, according to David Wheeler, microbiologist and senior research fellow at the Robens Institute at Surrey University. Full secondary treatment in a well operated plant can remove at least 99% of enteric bacteria, including salmonella, and 90% of enteroviruses—the remainder finding their way into the sea. The new directive does not make secondary treatment obligatory—primary treatment is acceptable if the receiving waters can accept the effluent without environmental damage—although the new treatment schemes will be designed so that the sea water meets the standards of the bathing water directive. Some debate, however, still remains over the microbiological standards in the directive, which many authorities consider need updating.

At sea over standards

Most countries interpret the standards in the bathing water

Sewage treatment

Nearly 90% of Britain's sewage is treated at land based sewage treatment works, which discharge effluent into rivers, estuaries, and eventually the sea.[13] Ten per cent is discharged direct into the sea, and the remainder is treated in septic tanks.

Preliminary treatment—Paper, cloth, sticks, and other objects are removed by screens. Grit is allowed to settle in special tanks.

Primary treatment—Solid matter is left to settle to the bottom of settlement tanks as sludge. This takes from two to six hours.

Secondary treatment—Biological treatment with micro-organisms is used to encourage the oxidation of organic matter. The resulting liquid passes through a further settlement tank, after which at least 95% of its organic load will have been removed. If of a specified standard the effluent can be discharged straight into a river, or can receive further treatment.

Tertiary treatment—This produces a clear liquid containing very little organic matter but a large quantity of faecal and other bacteria. These die off naturally and rapidly in the rivers and sea. Possible forms of tertiary treatment include pebble bed clarifiers, irrigation over grassland, sand filtration, and microstraining through fine steel fabric.

Sludge treatment—Sludge may be pumped direct from primary tanks into the sea if this is practicable. If not it undergoes biological or chemical treatment to remove pathogens or excess water, or both, and to reduce odour. This changes it from a foul brew to a brown sludge with an earthy odour. It may be dried into a solid cake if it is to be transported by land or sea any distance. Disposal of sludge at sea is to be phased out by 1998. Alternative disposal sites are on farmland (after treatment to reduce pathogens), in landfill sites, or by incineration.

directive to their own liking. According to the House of Commons Environment Committee, a tacit agreement exists between all members of the European Community, to ignore the standards for enterovirus and salmonella as the zero levels required are unobtainable.[1] The only mandatory standards are for total and faecal coliforms, which are used as indicators of contamination of the sea water by sewage.

As evidence linking minor illnesses with swimming in the sea mounts up, the importance of testing for viruses increases. Not only are viruses potentially responsible for many of the minor illnesses associated with sea bathing but they decay at a slower rate in the sea than bacteria and can cause infection at much lower doses. It may be that faecal streptococci, which have a longer survival time than coli-

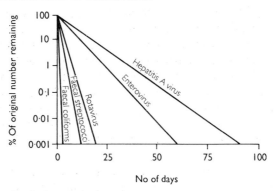

Typical survival characteristics of faecal bacteria and human enteric viruses in seawater[11]

forms, will emerge as a better indicator of sewage contamination in future (figure).

In the United States a dose response curve measuring degree of risk in terms of degree of exposure to pollution has been drawn up by the Environmental Protection Agency, based on the results of Cabelli's research. The United States is altogether more interventionist than Britain over its policy for coastal bathing. Beaches are actually closed when a certain number of samples fail to reach the predetermined standard.[1] One of the difficulties with closure is that beaches often fail because storms disperse sewage onshore. The water sampled from a beach taken at such a time will fail—even though no one would be tempted to bathe. The United States Environmental Protection Agency has not yet resolved the problem of when to open the beach again. The decision of whether or not the sea is too polluted to swim in is still left up to individuals in Britain—but increasingly they are being helped in their decision by the use of beach guides.

Beach guides

Beach guides have flourished in the past few years and the public is now faced with a seemingly ever increasing amount of information on which to base the decision whether to swim.

The local authority guide recommended by the Department of the Environment has attempted to provide comprehensive information to the public and not simply regurgitate the results of tests carried out by the National Rivers Authority. It provides some explanation about the quality of the bathing water by dividing beaches into three categories according to the quality of the sea water—excellent water quality (complying with the European Community guideline standards), good quality (complying with the mandatory standards), and poor quality (those which fail both the previous tests). But a survey carried out by the Marine Conservation Society earlier this year found that where the water was of poor quality the local authority was not interested in publicising any results. The society believes that compulsory guides are the only way to make the local authority scheme work.

The Marine Conservation Society's own guide, *The Good Beach Guide* (Ebury Press), is also based on the European Commission directive and has looked at more than 450 beaches in Britain. Most passed or marginally failed the mandatory guidelines, but only a few get its full four star rating for passing all tests at the guideline level.

The European Blue Flag Campaign was started in 1987 as part of the European Year of the Environment. In Britain it is supported by the Tidy Britain Group and the English Tourist Board with further help from the Department of the Environment, the National Rivers Authority, and the local authorities. The award is given annually and is valid for only one year. It requires compliance not only with water quality, as defined by the bathing water directive, but with the standard of the facilities on the beach, including cleanliness, provision of toilets, and parking. Last year 35 beaches were awarded a blue flag. Table II shows the results for Europe in 1991. There has been concern that, because water quality parameters and values vary from country

TABLE 2—*Blue flag campaign awards by country, 1991*

Country	No of beaches awarded a blue flag
Greece	178
Denmark	173
Spain	170
France	104
Portugal	96
Southern Ireland	65
Italy	55
Britain	35
Netherlands	30
Belgium	25
Germany	22

to country, the awarding of blue flags to beaches may not be on a strictly comparable basis.[8]

Golden starfish awards are related to the blue flag scheme and are being piloted in Britain and Greece. They are awarded to beautiful remote beaches which cannot satisfy the blue flag criteria because they are too isolated and little used. Golden starfish awards were given to 13 beaches in Britain in 1991.

Conclusion

Swimming in the sea is the most natural of recreations. It would be a sad day if its benefits were outweighed by the risk of becoming ill. Research is still growing, but the links between gastrointestinal and upper respiratory symptoms and swimming in sea water contaminated by sewage are now irrefutable. The recovery programme for beaches is long overdue, but at least some action is at last being taken. But before all beaches can be deemed safe from pollution, a commonsense approach is probably the most sensible—if the water

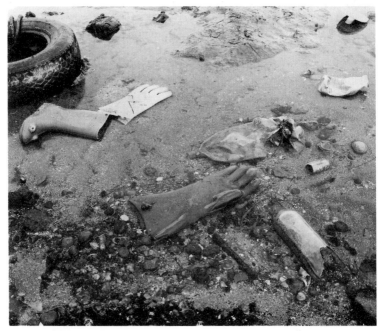

If a beach looks filthy, don't swim in the sea

looks filthy it would be unwise to swim in it. If all else fails join the crowds on the beaches with a blue flag, an "excellent" rating from the local authority, or a four star award from the *Good Beach Guide* and avoid the hazards of taking a dip.

1 House of Commons Environment Committee. *Pollution of beaches: fourth report.* London: HMSO, 1990.
2 Public Health Laboratory Service. Sewage contamination of coastal bathing waters in England and Wales: a bacteriological and epidemiological study. *J Hygiene* 1959;**57**:435-72.
3 Cabelli VJ, Dufour AP, McCabe LJ, Levin MA. Swimming—associated gastro-enteritis and water quality. *Am J Epidemiol* 1982;**115**:606-16.
4 Pike EB. *Phase 1 pilot study at Langland Bay.* London: Water Research Centre, 1990. (Department of Environment report 2518-M(P).)
5 Pike EB. *Health effects of sea bathing. Phase II studies at Ramsgate and Moreton, 1990.* London: Water Research Centre, 1991. (Department of Environment report 2736-M(P).)
6 Morris J. Sea survey continues. *Water Bulletin* 1991;**465**:7.
7 Balarajan R, Raleigh VS, Yuen P, Wheeler D, Machin D, Cartwright R. Health risks associated with bathing in sea water. *BMJ* 1991;**303**:144-5.
8 National Rivers Authority. *Bathing water quality in England and Wales—1990.* Bristol: NRA, 1991.
9 Dunlop JM. Blooming algae. *BMJ* 1991;**302**:671-2.
10 National Rivers Authority. *Toxic blue green algae.* London: NRA, 1990.
11 Wheeler D. On the beach. *Lab Practice* 1990;**39**:19-24.
12 Water Services Association. *Water information. Wastewater discharges to sea.* London: Water Services Association, 1991.
13 Hall C. *Running water.* London: Robertson McCarta, 1990.

Environmental radiation: a cause for concern

FIONA GODLEE

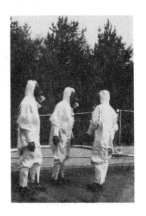

Radiation is an obvious focus for public concern. It is known to cause cancer and inspires anxiety because—unlike that other widely available carcinogen, cigarette smoke—it is beyond the individual's control. But is there evidence that radiation at levels encountered in the environment is dangerous to health?

Sources of radiation

Ionising radiation has always been part of our natural environment, being emitted from the earth's core and the solar system (box). It is only in the past few centuries that man has added to natural background radiation: underground mining has led to exposure from radioactive rocks; air and space travel have taken people closer to the sources of cosmic radiation; modern building technology has contributed to the accumulation of the radioactive gas radon in homes; and the discovery of x rays has spawned a whole industry of diagnostic and therapeutic radiology.[1]

The National Radiological Protection Board estimates that the average person in Britain receives a dose of radiation of 2·5 mSv each year. Of this, 87% comes from natural sources—over half from radon decay products in the home. Medical radiation contributes 12%. All other artificial sources—nuclear fall out, occupational exposure, and discharges from nuclear installations—account for about 1% of the total amount (fig 1).

Some basic physics

x Rays, γ rays, and α and β particles are emitted from unstable nuclei during radioactive decay. They are all forms of ionising radiation, so called because they possess sufficient energy to ionise atoms by removing electrons from them. Other forms of radiation—heat, light, radio waves, and microwaves—lack sufficient energy to do this and are therefore called non-ionising. α Particles, comprising two protons and two neutrons, are positively charged, heavy, and slow moving. They are emitted by uranium, thorium, and plutonium, and they ionise by dragging away electrons. β Particles, which are positive or negative electrons, are small and fast and less ionising than α particles. *x* Rays and γ rays are types of electromagnetic radiation. They are not charged but penetrate further than α and β particles. The biological effects of different types of radiation depend on the energy delivered per distance travelled, or the linear energy transfer (LET). α Particles (high linear energy transfer) have greater biological effects than β particles and γ rays (low linear energy transfer).

Measuring radioactivity

Bequerel (Bq)—a measure of the ionising activity of a sample; 1 Bq is one nuclear transformation per second.

Gray (Gy)—a measure of the amount of ionising energy absorbed by the body, or the absorbed dose; 1 Gy equals one joule of energy absorbed per kilogram of tissue. The gray has replaced the old rad: 1 Gy equals 100 rad.

Sieverts (Sv)—take into account the different linear energy transfer of different types of radiation. Multiplying the absorbed dose by one for β particles and 20 for α particles gives the dose equivalent in sieverts. The sievert has replaced the old rem: 1 Sv equals 100 rem.

The discovery of high levels of radon in homes in some areas of Britain has given the nuclear industry a chance to put its own contribution to environmental radiation into perspective and diverted public attention away from nuclear installations. But radon is a natural product of the environment; nuclear bombs and nuclear power are not. With the accident at Chernobyl and continuing anxiety about leukaemia clusters near nuclear plants in Britain, the industry's public relations officers are still hard pressed to reassure us that environmental radiation is safe.

Estimating the risks

There is almost no direct evidence that low doses of radiation

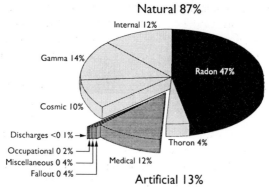

FIG 1 — *Contribution of different sources of radiation to annual average dose*[2]

(below 100 mSv) are dangerous to health.[3] But currently accepted mechanisms of causation of cancer are not consistent with the concept of a dose threshold, above which cancer will occur and below which there is no risk. It is therefore generally assumed that the risk from low dose radiation is so small that it is difficult to show epidemiologically.

Estimates of the risks from exposure to low doses of radiation are based on data from high dose exposure. These come from studies of survivors of the Japanese atomic bomb explosions, patients treated with radiotherapy, and workers in the nuclear industry.

Between 1950 and 1985 there were 340 excess deaths from cancer in a group of nearly 76 000 Japanese survivors.[4] There have also been reports of short stature, reduced intelligence quotient (IQ), and increased rates of cancer later in life in their children.[5] The dose of radiation to which these survivors were exposed has been calculated, and dose response curves for induction of cancer have been drawn up. By extrapolating the curve back towards zero the effects of radiation at low doses can be estimated.

But there are problems with this approach. Firstly, backward extrapolation along a dose response curve assumes that the relation between the dose and the response is linear. If the relation was instead quadratic or linear quadratic, as some models suggest (fig 2),[6] the risks from radiation at low doses would be lower than predicted from the linear curve.

Secondly, the calculated doses received by the survivors are only estimates. They are based on such things as an individual's distance from the explosion and the shielding effect of intervening buildings. As a result of new evidence from Japan these estimates have recently been extensively revised, suggesting that the risks of cancer from radiation may be three to four times higher than was previously thought.

A third problem is the difference in the nature of the exposure. The doses inflicted by the bombing of Hiroshima and Nagasaki—in many cases over 200 mGy—are 10 times the levels being considered in low dose chronic exposure and were inflicted over a short period. Risk estimates must also take into account the fact that extrapolating from the so called "high dose, high dose rate" exposure will further underestimate the risk of cancer from "low dose, low dose rate" environmental radiation.[6]

A better basis for assessing risk from low dose chronic exposure may be studies on workers at nuclear installations. Occupational exposure is lower than that from the atomic bomb explosions—with average cumulative exposures of 1·4 and 7·8 mSv in two recent

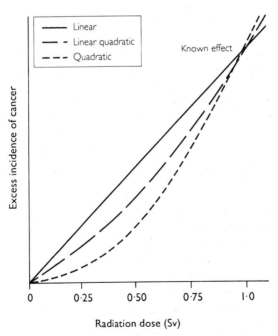

FIG 2—*Dose response curves for linear, quadratic, and linear quadratic models*[6]

studies[7][8]—and is inflicted over a longer period. In addition, each worker's exposure is monitored by the wearing of film badges which record the cumulative dose of external radiation. These studies have found small increases in death rates from cancers such as leukaemia, multiple myeloma, lung cancer, and secondary cancers.[7][9] At the same time some cancers—for example, Hodgkin's disease and liver cancer—occur less often than expected.

In 1985 Beral et al found a significant increase in relative risk of prostatic cancer in workers from the British Atomic Energy Authority; the increase was strongly related to radiation dose.[10] In a second study in 1988, this time on workers in the Atomic Weapons Establishment, the increased risk of prostatic cancer was less evident, except in those workers who were also exposed to internal radiation from ingesting radionuclides such as polonium, uranium, and tritium.[8] Beral et al concluded that the increase in prostatic cancer was unlikely to be due to external radiation alone. Other studies—for example, one of survivors of atomic bomb explosions[11] and a recent one of over 95 000 British radiation workers[9]—have failed to find any effect on mortality from cancer of the prostate.

The risk estimates for low dose radiation remain highly uncertain and are constantly being revised. The 1990 estimate from the International Commission on Radiological Protection—0·05 cancer deaths per Sv for a population of all ages—is based on a linear, no threshold model and incorporates a "dose rate effectiveness factor" to correct for chronic exposure.[12] It is four times higher than the last estimate in 1977.[13]

Leukaemia clusters

In 1983 a Yorkshire Television programme, *Windscale: the Nuclear Laundry*, alleged that emissions from the nuclear reprocessing plant in west Cumbria had caused a local increase in the incidence of leukaemia in children. Reports subsequently confirmed the cluster around Windscale (renamed Sellafield in an attempt to shed unhappy associations) and showed other clusters near nuclear installations at Dounreay in Scotland and at Aldermaston and Burghfield in Berkshire.[14-16] Sellafield—the only reprocessing plant out of the four installations—discharges much the highest level of radiation into the environment and is associated with the largest excess risk of childhood leukaemia: a 10-fold increase in the number of cases over 30 years compared with a twofold increase near the other three installations.

Analysis of data from nuclear installations throughout England and Wales showed similar trends.[17] Between 1969 and 1978 mortality from all leukaemias in those aged 0–24 years was 15% higher in districts near nuclear installations than in matched control districts, and mortality from lymphoid leukaemia was 21% higher.[18] Although small by comparison with the 10-fold excess around Sellafield, these figures reached significance because of the large numbers being studied. The Committee on Medical Aspects of Radiation in the Environment, an independant advisory body, concluded that the clusters, especially the one around Sellafield, are unlikely to be due to chance.[16] The reason for the clustering, however, remains a mystery.

The committee found little evidence to incriminate radiation. The doses that the children are thought to have received are, says the committee, far too low to explain the increase in incidence. Samples of bone marrow from 1 year old children in Britain have shown an average dose from background radiation of about 990 μSv. The additional dose to the bone marrow of 1 year olds living near Sellafield is only 170 μSv and near Dounreay only 4·5 μSv.[19] These data have been the mainstay of arguments from the nuclear industry against any association between discharges from nuclear plants and leukaemia clusters.

Further evidence against environmental radiation as the major cause of the clusters comes from a study that found a similar excess risk of leukaemia in areas where nuclear installations were planned but either never built or built after the data on mortality had been gathered.[20] This implies that radiation is not responsible and that potential and existing nuclear sites share some as yet unrecognised risk factor for leukaemia. Other explanations for the clusters need to be examined.

One alternative explanation, though not widely accepted, is that childhood leukaemia is a rare consequence of some as yet unidentified infection.[21-23] The main proponent of this theory, Dr Leo Kinlen, director of the Cancer Epidemiology Unit in Oxford, cites the fact that infectious causes, in the form of specific viruses, are well established for several animal leukaemias and for adult T cell leukaemia. In addition, he believes that the pattern of leukaemia in the areas studied fits the model of an epidemic; starting in the 1950s, reaching a peak in the late 1970s, and then dying away again. Kinlen suggests that building nuclear installations in isolated areas provides the ideal set up for an infectious epidemic. People who have previously remained unexposed to an infectious agent are susceptible to infection. Mixing with a population of exposed individuals will ensure a large dose of the agent and increase the chances of infection. The infectious theory is likely to remain speculative unless a specific agent is identified.

Meanwhile, a new hypothesis—that a man's exposure to radiation is associated with an increased risk of leukaemia in his children—has shifted the spotlight back on to the nuclear industry. The hypothesis was formulated during analysis of the Sellafield data.[24] The risk of leukaemia was found to be raised if a child's father had been employed at Sellafield and was highest when the father's cumulative exposure exceeded 100 mSv or when he was exposed to more than 10 mSv in the six months before the child's conception. The study found no link with direct environmental exposure to the child from, for example, using local beaches or eating seafood or home grown vegetables.

One much quoted animal study lends limited support to the idea that childhood cancers might be caused by previous parental exposure. Irradiation of male mice has been shown to increase the risk of leukaemia (and lung cancer) in their offspring.[25] The study by Gardner et al[24] has proved more difficult for the nuclear industry to poke holes in than previous work. This is not only because of its statistical rigour but also because, by moving away from the idea of a direct effect of radiation, it may explain the discrepancy between Sellafield's small contribution to local children's overall dose of environmental radiation and the 10-fold increase in the risk of childhood leukaemia. Gardner's findings are, however, based on a small number of cases on which a large number of tests were performed and must therefore be considered as preliminary.

Other studies have found no effect from previous parental exposure. Children of survivors of the atomic bomb explosions at Hiroshima and Nagasaki have not shown an increased risk of cancer.[26 27] And a case-control study of children with leukaemia and lymphoma in the area around Dounreay found no association with the fathers' exposure to radiation.[28] The Japanese data, however, deal with acute massive exposure to radiation and may not be relevant to chronic low dose exposure; and although the Dounreay study failed to confirm Gardner's hypothesis, the small number of cases meant that it did not have the power to refute it. More work and larger studies are needed to test the hypothesis.

Medical radiation

Medicine is the largest source of manmade radiation. It also offers the greatest scope for reducing the dose of radiation delivered to the population.[29] The doses now used are, however, small relative to background radiation, and any excess risk is difficult to detect.

The early days of medical radiation were characterised by much misguided enthusiasm. Ringworm, acne, birthmarks, bursitis, and sinusitis were among the benign conditions treated with deep radiation therapy. The scalps of more than 10 000 children in Israel, and a similar number in New York, were irradiated for ringworm between 1949 and 1960 with the intention of making the hair fall out so that the skin could be more effectively treated.[30] It was only in the 1960s that an awareness of the potential dangers began to dawn. Studies in America comparing irradiated and non-irradiated children infested with ringworm have shown a sixfold increase in cancers of the thyroid as well as smaller increases in brain cancers and leukaemia.[31][32]

High doses of radiation were also delivered to induce menopause in patients with menorrhagia and in mass screening for tuberculosis. Tuberculosis was, however, a rampant killer in the days before antibiotics, and early diagnosis was the only means of attack. In Britain the radiological vogue was for treating ankylosing spondylitis.

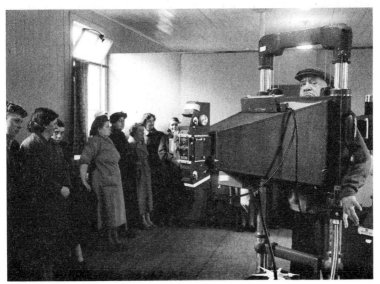

Mass screening: justified in the days before antibiotics but not now

113

A study of 14 111 patients with the disease who were given a single course of x ray treatment between 1935 and 1954 showed a two thirds increase in mortality from all causes and a nearly fivefold excess of deaths from leukaemia.[33] In the past 20 years the doses used in medicine have been greatly reduced, and radiation has been increasingly reserved for treating malignant conditions and for diagnostic purposes.

Diagnostic radiology offers perhaps the only piece of direct evidence that low doses of radiation are a risk to health. This comes from some studies performed in the 1950s which showed that children born to women who were irradiated during pregnancy had an increased incidence of cancer.[34] As a result of such findings, the 10 day rule—which states that women of reproductive age should have x ray examinations only within 10 days of the start of their last menstrual period—has been adopted in Britain. It remains controversial, however, and is not used by the American College of Radiology. The International Committee on Radiological Protection now recommends that there is no need to limit exposure until after the fourth week of pregnancy.[35]

In Britain diagnostic medical x rays comprise almost nine tenths of the total collective dose of radiation from all manmade sources.[29] The table shows the estimated risk of cancer from different types of radiography. About 25 million x ray examinations are performed each year in the NHS, one third of them chest examinations. France and the United States perform about twice as many x ray examinations as Britain per head of population, and Japan averages four x ray

Estimates of risk of fatal cancer from single x ray examinations of different types[29]

x Ray examination	Average lifetime risk of fatal cancer (per million)
Skull	2-7
Chest	0·7-2
Thoracic spine	15-40
Lumbar spine	30-100
Abdomen	20-60
Pelvis	15-55
Intravenous urography	60-200
Barium meal	50-170
Barium enema	100-350

examinations per person per year (National Radiological Protection Board, personal communication).

Many of these investigations are unnecessary. According to a recent report from the Joint Working Party of the National Radiological Protection Board and the Royal College of Radiologists, at least one fifth of all x ray examinations performed in Britain are not clinically helpful,[36] and in one study a third of patients sent to an orthopaedic clinic in Scotland had to have repeat examinations because their original films were not provided by the general practitioner.[37] The National Radiological Protection Board estimates that 3-15% of x ray examinations are repeated because of unsatisfactory results at the first attempt.[29] The radiation from unnecessary diagnostic irradiation amounts to 7500 man Sv and could be responsible for 100-250 of Britain's 160 000 yearly deaths from cancer.

Reducing the dose

The contribution to environmental radiation from radiography could be tackled by reducing both the number of investigations and the dose delivered with each one. The Royal College of Radiologists and the National Radiological Protection Board have recently issued new guidelines on the use of routine radiological investigations.[36] Preoperative chest radiography is only indicated in patients about to undergo cardiac or pulmonary surgery or in whom there is a strong suspicion of malignancy or tuberculosis. Skull radiography should not be performed routinely after head injury, and employment related screening is discouraged. In 1983 an estimated 140 000 "employment related" chest radiographs were taken in Britain, delivering an annual collective dose of about 5 man Sv. They should be taken only when clinically justified—for example, in workers from countries where tuberculosis is endemic.

These can only ever be guidelines. The Royal College of Radiologists recognises that imposing absolute limits on the amount of radiation to which a patient can be exposed would be impossible. Acute medical emergencies will always take precedence over the long term risks to the patient from additional exposure to x rays. But the college is creating an atmosphere in which clinicians must justify their requests for radiological investigations.

Additional restraint is being encouraged in screening for treatable diseases. The Forrest report recommends that mammography should be reserved for women aged 50 to 64.[38] Those aged 65 and over should be screened only on demand. The position of women under the age of 50 remains controversial, but in the absence of strong evidence of benefit the advice is to screen only those with a history of premenopausal breast cancer in a first degree relative.

As well as reducing the number of radiological investigations there is scope for reducing the dose administered with each one. Simply by making optimum use of existing technology the average radiation dose to patients could be halved.[36]

Proper use of gonad shields would reduce the risk of severe hereditary disease. A survey in 1980 found that gonad shields were not being used as often as they should be, especially in children.[39] They should be used in all patients of or below reproductive age.

Computed tomography delivers relatively high doses of radiation, and doses have increased rather than decreased as technology has advanced. This is because the speed of imaging has increased dramatically, leading to a rise in the number of slices imaged on each patient. At the same time little progress has been made towards reducing the dose of radiation given with each slice. Computed tomography comprises only 2% of x ray examinations in Britain but contributes 20% of the effective collective radiation dose.[36] Routine abdominal computed tomography delivers an effective dose of 9 mSv—as much as a barium enema.

The future of diagnostic imaging may be radiation free thanks to the arrival of nuclear magnetic resonance. But this form of imaging also has its limitations. At the moment it is expensive and there are practical problems in encasing patients inside the magnet. There have also recently been some anxieties about its safety in certain patients.[40]

Radon

The biggest contribution to natural radiation comes from radon, a colourless, odourless gas given off by uranium. Granite contains uranium and emits radon into the atmosphere, especially in areas where the rock is heavily fractured. Radon emits α particles as it decays to radioactive polonium, lead, and bismuth. These "radon daughters," α emitters in their own right, are then inhaled.

In the past uranium miners were heavily exposed to radon, and studies have shown them to be at increased risk of lung cancer.[41 42] People living in areas well endowed with granite are also exposed, especially since modern building techniques have improved insulation in houses. In Pennsylvania an engineer at a nuclear power station set off radiation alarms as he arrived at work. His house, well insulated and built on ground rich in granite, was found to have an indoor radon level of 100 000 Bq/m³. Higher levels have since been recorded in both America and Britain.

The United States Environmental Protection Agency has set 150 Bq/m³ as the concentration of radon at which remedial action should be taken. It estimates the lifetime risk of fatal lung cancer from exposure at this level to be 2·4%-9%. On this basis 5000 to 20 000 of the 130 000 annual deaths from lung cancer in the United States could be attributed to exposure to radon.

In Britain the action level for existing houses has recently been halved from 400 to 200 Bq/m³ in response to the National Radiological Protection Board's reappraisal of the risk from radon in homes.[43] An estimated 100 000 houses in the United Kingdom currently exceed this level, most of them in Devon and Cornwall. The average concentration of radon in homes across the country is estimated at 20 Bq/m³. This confers an average lifetime risk of lung cancer of 0·3%, and implies that one in 20 lung cancers in Britain (about 2000 cases a year) may be due to radon exposure at home.[43] Radon in homes in Britain is measured by the National Radiological Protection Board on behalf of the Department of the Environment. Surveys are free if, because of the locality, the board considers it likely that the radon level will be raised or if the house is in an area where little is known about radon levels. Otherwise the householder is charged £29.60 plus value added tax.

Advice on remedial action from the Building Research Establishment aims at preventing radon from entering houses.[44] The air pressure inside houses tends to be lower than outside because of the effect of wind and temperature. As a result, soil gas containing radon is drawn up into the house. This can be prevented by drawing air from beneath the floor with an extractor fan. According to the Building Research Establishment, the cost of such remedial action would be £500-£1500.

It is important, however, to stress that at the moment there is little direct evidence that radon at levels found in houses causes lung cancer. Current risk estimates are based on extrapolation from the known effects on uranium miners and, like those based on the atomic bomb survivors, they assume a linear, no threshold relation between the dose of radon and the incidence of lung cancer. Estimates are corrected for the differences between the miners—all adult men performing heavy physical tasks breathing at high rates in a dust laden atmosphere—and the population at large.

Another factor that must be corrected for is smoking. Most of the miners on whom risk estimates have been based were heavy smokers. Studies that take this into account have led to the conclusion that smoking increases the carcinogenic effects of radon. The lifetime risk of exposure to radon for smokers is estimated to be 10 times that for non-smokers.

This has led to controversy over whether non-smokers are at any increased risk of lung cancer from low doses of radon. A study in Colorado of 516 non-smoking uranium miners found only a small excess of lung cancers.[45] This, in concert with the other uncertainties, prompted the authors of a recent review to suggest that the risks of radon at low dose have been overstated. They concluded that there is insufficient evidence to justify the National Radiological Protection Board's proposals for remedial action in homes.[46] The board says, however, that this review does not reflect the international scientific consensus.

Conclusion

The radiation story is far from complete. Risk estimates for radiation exposure are founded on shifting ground. If there is an excess risk from environmental radiation it remains undetected by current techniques and is therefore likely to be extremely small. Routine emissions from modern nuclear installations and from weapons testing seem to add little to the overall risks. But the nuclear industry still has a grave responsibility to protect its workers and their children from the effects of radiation and prevent the potentially devastating damage to health from nuclear accidents like the fire at Chernobyl. The effects of radiation on the body are cumulative, and whatever the source it makes sense to limit exposure when possible. Controlling the use of radiation in medicine offers great scope for preventing unnecessary death and illness.

1 Caufield C. *Multiple exposures—chronicles of the radiation age.* London: Secker and Warburg, 1989.
2 National Radiological Protection Board. *Living with radiation.* 4th ed. Chilton: NRPB, 1989.
3 Sumner D. Low level radiation—how dangerous is it? *Medicine and War* 1990;6: 112-9.

4 Beebe GW, Kato H, Land CE. Studies of the mortality of A bomb survivors. 6. Mortality and radiation dose, 1950-74. *Radiation Research* 1978;**75**:136-201.

5 Yoshimoto Y. Cancer risk among children of atomic bomb survivors. *JAMA* 1990;**264**:596-600.

6 Sumner D, Wheldon T, Watson W. *Radiation risks: an evaluation*. 3rd ed. Glasgow: Tarragon Press, 1991.

7 Wing S, Shy CM, Wood JL, Wolf S, Cragle DL, Frome EL. Mortality among workers at Oak Ridge National Laboratory. *JAMA* 1991;**265**:1397-402.

8 Beral V, Fraser P, Carpenter L, Booth M, Brown A, Rose G. Mortality of employees of the Atomic Weapons Establishment, 1951-82. *BMJ* 1988;**297**: 757-70.

9 Kendall G, Muirhead CR, MacGibbon BH, O'Hagan JA, Conquest AJ, Goodill AA, *et al*. Mortality and occupational exposure to radiation: first analysis of the National Registry for Radiation Workers. *BMJ* 1992;**304**: 220-5.

10 Beral V, Inskip H, Fraser P, Booth M, Coleman D, Rose G. Mortality of employees of the United Kingdom Atomic Energy Authority, 1946-1979. *BMJ* 1985;**291**: 440-7.

11 Shimizu Y, Kato H, Schull WJ, Preston DL, Fujita S, Pierce DA. Life span study report 11. Part 1. Comparison of risk coefficients for site-specific cancer mortality based on the DS86 and T65DR shielded Kerma and Organ doses. *Radiation Effects Research Foundation Technical Report Series* 1987; No 12:1-56.

12 International Commission on Radiological Protection. *Recommendations of the ICRP*. Oxford: ICRP, 1990.

13 International Commission on Radiological Protection. Recommendations of the ICRP 1977. *Ann ICRP* 1978:1.

14 Independent Advisory Group. *Investigation of the possible increased incidence of cancer in west Cumbria*. London: HMSO, 1984. (Black report.)

15 Committee on Medical Aspects of Radiation in the Environment. *Second report. Investigation of the possible increased incidence of leukaemia in young people near the Dounreay nuclear establishment, Caithness, Scotland*. London: HMSO, 1988.

16 Committee on Medical Aspects of Radiation in the Environment. *Third report. Report on the incidence of childhood cancer in the west Berkshire and north Hampshire area, in which are situated the Atomic Weapons Research Establishment, Aldermaston, and the Royal Ordnance Factory, Burghfield*. London: HMSO, 1989.

17 Forman D, Cook-Mozafarri P, Darby S, Davey G, Stratton I, Doll R, *et al*. Cancer near nuclear installations. *Nature* 1987;**329**:499-505.

18 Cook-Mozaffari PJ, Darby SC, Doll R. Geographical variation in mortality from leukaemia and other cancers in England and Wales, 1959-1980. *Office of Population Censuses and Surveys Studies on Medical and Population Subjects*. No 51. London: HMSO, 1987.

19 Stapher FK, Clarke RH, Duncan KP. *The risk of childhood leukaemia near nuclear establishments*. Chilton: National Radiological Protection Board, 1988. (NRPB-R215.)

20 Cook-Mozaffari P, Darby S, Doll R. Cancer near potential sites of nuclear installations. *Lancet* 1989;ii:1145-7.

21 Kinlen LJ. Evidence for an infective cause of childhood leukaemia: comparison of a Scottish new town with nuclear reprocessing sites in Britain. *Lancet* 1988;ii: 1323-7.

22 Kinlen LJ, Clarke K, Hudson C. Evidence from population mixing in British new towns 1946-85 of an infective basis of childhood leukaemia. *Lancet* 1990;ii: 577-82.

23 Kinlen LJ, Hudson C. Childhood leukaemia and poliomyelitis in relation to military encampments in England and Wales in the period of national military service, 1950-63. *BMJ* 1991;**303**:1357-62.

24 Gardner MJ, Snee MP, Hall AJ, Powell CA, Downes S, Terrell JD. Results of case-control study of leukaemia and lymphoma among young people near Sellafield nuclear plant in west Cumbria. *BMJ* 1990;**300**:423-34.

25 Nomura T. Parental exposure to *x* rays and chemicals induces heritable tumours and anomalies in mice. *Nature* 1982;**296**:575-7.

26 Ishimaru T, Ishimaru M, Mikami M. *Leukaemia incidence among individuals exposed in utero, children of atomic bomb survivors and their controls, Hiroshima and Nagasaki, 1945-79.* Hiroshima: Radiation Effects Research Foundation, 1981. (RERF technical report 11-81.)

27 Yoshimoto Y, Neel JV, Schull WJ. *Frequency of malignant tumours during the first two decades of life in the offspring (F1) of atomic bomb survivors.* Hiroshima: Radiation Effects Research Foundation, 1990. (RERF technical report 4-90.)

28 Urquhart JD, Black RJ, Muirhead MJ, Sharp L, Maxwell M, Eden OB, *et al.* Case-control study of leukaemia and non-Hodgkins lymphoma in children in Caithness near the Dounreay nuclear installation. *BMJ* 1990;**302**:687-92.

29 National Radiological Protection Board. *Patient dose reduction in diagnostic radiology.* Vol 1. No 3. Chilton: NRPB, 1990.

30 Ron E, Modan B. Benign and malignant thyroid neoplasms after childhood irradiation for tinea capitis. *J Natl Cancer Inst* 1980;**65**:7-11.

31 Modan B, Ron E, Werner W. Thyroid cancer following scalp irradiation. *Therapeutic Radiology* 1977;**123**:741-4.

32 Modan B, Baidatz D, Mart H. Radiation induced head and neck tumours. *Lancet* 1974;i:277-9.

33 Smith PG, Doll R. Mortality among patients with ankylosing spondylitis after a single treatment course with *x* rays. *BMJ* 1982;**284**:449-60.

34 Stewart A, Kneale GW. Radiation dose effects in relation to obstetric *x* rays and childhood cancers. *Lancet* 1970;i:1185-7.

35 International Committee on Radiological Protection. The 1983 Washington meeting of ICRP. *Radiological Protection Bulletin* 1984;**57**:11.

36 National Radiological Protection Board and Royal College of Radiologists. Patient dose reduction in diagnostic radiology. Report of the Royal College of Radiologists and the National Radiological Protection Board. *Documents of the National Radiological Protection Board* 1990;1(3).

37 Bransby-Zachary MAP, Sutherland GR. Unnecessary *x* ray examinations. *BMJ* 1989;**298**:1294.

38 Report of a DHSS working group. *Report to the health ministers of England, Wales, Scotland, and Northern Ireland. Breast cancer screening.* London: HMSO, 1986. (Forrest report).

39 Wall BF, Fisher ES, Shrimpton PC, Rae S. *Current levels of gonadal irradiation from a selection of routine diagnostic x ray examinations in Great Britain.* London: HMSO, 1980. (NRPB-R105.)

40 National Radiological Protection Board. Board statement on clinical magnetic resonance diagnostic procedures. *Documents of the National Radiological Protection Board, 1991.*

41 International Commission on Radiological Protection. Lung cancer risk from indoor exposure to radon daughters. ICRP publication 50. *Ann ICRP* 1987;**17** (No 1).

42 Committee on the Biological Effects of Ionising Radiation. *Health risks of radon and other internally deposited alpha emitters (Beir IV).* Washington, DC: National Radiological Commission, 1988.

43 National Radiological Protection Board. Board statement on radon in homes. *Documents of the National Radiological Protection Board* 1990;1(1).

44 Department of the Environment. *The householder's guide to radon.* 2nd ed. London: DoE, 1990.

45 Roscoe RJ, Steenland K, Halperin WE. Lung cancer mortality among non-smoking uranium miners exposed to radon daughters. *JAMA* 1989;**262**:629-33.
46 Bowie C, Bowie SH. Radon and health. *Lancet* 1991;**337**:409-13.

Index

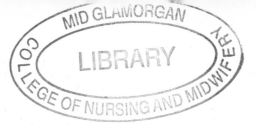

acid gases, and air pollution 47
acid rain 2, 3, 47
Africa
  bicycles 70
  food imports 10
  population growth 14
aging and hearing loss 77
aid programmes 15-6
AIDS epidemic 14
air pollution 44-64
  control 60-2
  particulate 44, 47, 62
    and allergy 56
  sulphurous 44-7
allergy, air pollution and 55-6
aluminium in water 90-1
Alzheimer's disease 90
ankylosing spondylitis, radiation and
  113-14
Antarctic, ozone layer over 27-8
Aral Sea 11
Asia
  bicycles 69
  population growth 14
asthma, air pollution and 55-6
audiometric screening 78
Australia
  deaths from asthma 56
  melanoma 29
  skin cancer 29

Badenoch, Sir John 90
bathing water, quality 103
beach guides 102-4
benzene 59-60, 62
bicycles 69-70
bladder cancer, transport workers 58
blue flags 103
boilermakers' deafness 75
bottled water 5, 90
Boyd, David 37
Britain
  beaches 99
  bicycles 70
  car journeys 69
  carbon dioxide emissions 61

Britain (continued)
  chlorofluorocarbons policy 32
  complaints about noise 79
  cryptosporidiosis 89
  deaths from asthma 56
  distances travelled by car 66
  emissions policy 24
  gastric cancer 91
  hearing damage 74, 77
  public transport 69
  reducing power station emissions 60
  risks of sea bathing 96-8
  road accidents 65
bronchitis, air pollution and 45

Cabelli, Victor 96
Camelford, water supply accident 85, 91
Canada, deaths from asthma 56
cancer
  air pollution and 57-9
  bladder 58
  low dose radiation and 108
  lung 58, 116-17
  melanoma 3, 29-31
  prostatic 110
  skin 3, 28-9, 31, 32
  x ray examinations and 115
carbon dioxide 5, 19
  concentrations 2
  emissions 3, 24, 61
cardiovascular disease, and hardness of
  water 92
cars
  disincentives to driving 71
  growth rate in ownership 66
  and rich-poor gap 67
  see also vehicles
catalytic converters 61, 62
cataracts, and ultraviolet light 31
Chadwick, Edwin 37
chemical contaminants in water 89, 90- 2
chest infections, air pollution and 45
childhood cancers 58
  previous parental radiation exposure
    112
China

China (*continued*)
    air pollution 48
    cycling 70, 71
    family planning 16
chlorofluorocarbons 1-2, 5
    and and ozone 27
    United Nations agreement 32
Clean Air Act 47
climatic change 19-26
Clinton Davis, Stanley 42
coal *see* fossil fuels
coal, brown 48
coliforms 101
Committee on Medical Aspects of
        Radiation in the Environment 111
company cars 67
computed tomography 116
contraceptives, distribution 16-7
crops, damage to 11
cryptosporidiosis 89-90
cyanobacteria 99
cycling 66, 69-70
cycling helmets 66
Czechoslovakia, air pollution and disease
        48-9

damage, environmental, reversal 5-6
Davis, Adrian 75, 77
deafness, noise at work and 75
deforestation 3, 11, 19, 24
demographic trap 15
Denmark
    cycling 70
    gastric cancer 91
desertification 11
developing countries *see* Third World
dialysis dementia 90
diesel fumes 47, 57, 61-2
dioxin 39-40
disasters, natural 22
discos, effect on hearing 75-6
disease
    noise and 82-3
    waste disposal and 89
    see also specific diseases
disinfection, of water 87
doctors, role of 5
Doll, Sir Richard 57, 59
drinking water *see* water

electrostatic precipitators 60
Elwood, Peter 83
emissions, stabilising 24
energy consumption 1

Environment Protection Act 80
Europe, eastern, environmental recovery
        49-50
European Blue Flag Campaign 103
European Commission directives
    bathing water 98
    drinking water 88
    municipal waste water 100
exposure, estimation of 5

faecal contamination of water 89
family planning 5, 15, 16-7
Farman, Joe 27
fertility, decreasing 12, 13, 17
fly tipping 38
fogs, winter 4, 44, 45
food crisis 5
food production 9-12
fossil fuels 24
    brown coal 48
    consumption 20
France
    beaches 99
    deaths from asthma 56
    x ray examinations 114

gastric cancer, and nitrate 91
gastrointestinal symptoms, sea bathing
        and 98
Germany
    chlorofluorocarbons policy 32
    clinical waste 37
    reducing emissions 24
    reducing power station emissions 60
    traffic calming measures 71
Germany, eastern, air pollution 48
global warming 2, 3, 19-24
    and health 20-2
golden starfish awards 104
gonad shields 116
grain production 5, 9
    sea level rise and 23
green cards 92
greenhouse effect 20
    see also global warming
greenhouse gases 2, 19
groundwater, contamination of 85-6
guidelines, radiological examinations 115

Hanna, Judith 72
hardness of water 92
hay fever 55, 56
Health and Safety Executive 78
healthy worker effect 58

hearing loss,
  noise induced 74-8
  prevention 77
Hong Kong, public transport 69
Hungary, gastric cancer 91

immunosuppression, and ultraviolet B
  31
India
  soil erosion 10-1
  sulphur dioxide emissions 48
industrialised countries, population
  growth 13
industry
  effects on environment 53-64
  emissions 2
  wastes 40-1
infant mortality 15
intelligence, and lead 91
International Panel on Climate Change 3
Ireland, beaches 99
irrigation 11-2
Italy, gastric cancer 91

Japan
  acidic gases 48
  atomic bomb survivors,
    and cancer 113
    and radiation exposure 108
  catalytic converters 61
  reducing power station emissions 60
  x ray examination 114

King, Maurice 15
Kinlen, Leo 111

land, agricultural,
  contaminated by waste 41
  loss of 23
landfill, contamination of groundwater 86
  gas 41
  sites 40-1
Langland Bay studies 97
lead
  in air and blood 61
  in water 91-2
legislation
  air pollution 47
  catalytic converters 61
  chlorofluorocarbons 32
  ground water 41
  noise 78
  ozone 55
  waste disposal 36

legislation (continued)
  water impurities 87
leukaemia clusters 110-2
London
  1952 fog 4, 44, 45, 46
  car ownership 67
  clinical wastes 35
  cycle routes 71
  traffic 67
  water 93
London Cycling Campaign 66
London Waste Regulation Authority 36,
  37
Los Angeles
  benzene 60
  land use for traffic 67
  mortality in heat waves 21
Love Canal 41
lung cancer
  diesel exhaust and 58
  radon and 116-7
lung function, ozone and 55, 56

McCaig, R H 78
mammography 115-6
Marine Conservation Society 103
Marriot, Liz 66, 71, 72
Matthews, Peter 88
media, and water pollution issues 88,
  92-3
melanoma, malignant 3, 29-31
methaemoglobinaemia 91
microbiological contaminants in water
  89-90
microbiological standards, bathing water
  100
migration 13, 14
Montreal accord 5, 31
Moreton Beach studies 98
mortality, temperature and 21

National Radiological Protection Board
  117
National Rivers Authority 98
Netherlands,
  beaches 99
  cycling 70, 71
  reducing emissions 24, 60
neurotoxicity, and aluminium 90
Nigeria, distribution of contraceptives 17
nitrate in water 91
nitric oxide 53
nitrogen dioxide, vehicle emissions 3, 4
noise 74-93
  annoyance 78-81

noise *(continued)*
  measuring 75
  positive effects 81
  risk levels for hearing 74-5
  susceptibility 77
  tolerance 79
Noise Abatement Society 80
Noise at Work Regulations 78
nuclear energy 3
nuclear magnetic resonance 116
nuclear workers, and radiation exposure 109

ozone
  depletion 27-33
    and health 28-31
  formation 27
  ground level 4, 20, 53-5
  layer 2, 3
    effect on crops 23
    predictions 28

Packham, Ronald 88
Parr, Doug 32
particulate traps 61, 62
pea soupers 4, 45
personal stereos, effect on hearing 76
pesticides in water 5, 88, 92
Pesticides Incident Monitoring Unit 92
phytoplankton 2
Pike, Edmond 97
Poland, air pollution and disease 48, 49
population growth 1
  and grain production 23
  control 5, 9-18
  rate 12-3
power stations, emissions 60
pregnancy, *x* rays and 114
prostatic cancer, radiation and 110
psychiatric problems, noise and 81-2
public transport 69

radiation 106-21
  dose reduction 115-6
  leaks 3
  low dose, risk estimates 110
  measuring exposure 108-10
  medical 106, 113-5
  sources 106-7, 108
radioactivity, measuring 107
radiography, cancer risk 114
radon 106, 107, 116-8
  smoking and 118
Ramsgate Sands studies 98

recycling schemes 42
refugees, environmental 23
regulations, waste disposal 40
reservoirs 86
Rice, Chris 76, 78
ringworm, radiation and 113
risk compensation 66
river pollution 86
road accidents 65-6
road building, effect on traffic 68
road traffic 53-64, 66-7, 80
  emissions 61-2
  reduction 63
  see also vehicles
Robinson, Douglas 74, 77
Royal National Institute for the Deaf 76
rubbish collection 37

Scandinavia, reducing power station emissions 60
scrubbers 60
sea bathing, health risks 95-8
sea level, rise in 22-3
Sellafield 110, 112
seroconversion, and clinical wastes 34-5
sewage
  contaminating sea water 5, 95
  treatment 99-100, 101
sharps injuries 35
skin cancer 3
  and immunosuppression 31
  malignant melanomas 29-31
  non-melanocytic 29-9
  prevention 32
sleep disturbance, noise and 80-1
smog, photochemical 4, 44, 53
smoking, and effects of radon 118
Snow, John 89
soil erosion 10-1
solar heat 19
Soviet Union, emissions policy 24
Sri Lanka, family planning 16
Stansfield, Stephen 82
streptococci, in sea water 101
sulphur dioxide 44
  vehicle emissions 4
sunbathing, and melanoma 29
Sweden
  waste 40, 41
  waterborne disease 89
swimming,
  in inland water 99
  in sea water 95-9
Switzerland, cancer 59

tall stack policy 47, 60
tap water 5, 85, 90, 93
technical fixes, vehicle emissions 61-2
temperature, and mortality 21
temperature rise *see* global warming
10 day rule 114
Third World 5
 aid to 15-6
 air pollution 48
 cycling 69
 environmental recovery 50
 exploitation of land 9
 family size 17
 food production 12
 global warming and 24
 health of infants 15-6
 and mistakes of industrialised world
  17, 50
 population growth 13, 17
  control 14-5
 road accidents 65
Thompson, Shirley 82
tinnitus 76-7
Townend, Bill 38
toxins 5
traffic
 average speed 66-7
 emissions 61-2
  reduction 63
 noise 80
 see also vehicles
transport 65-73
 public 69
 use of 68
 see also road traffic, vehicles
Transport and Health Study Group 71
transport strategy 71, 72
tropical diseases 21
tuberculosis 113

ultraviolet light 2, 11, 27, 28, 29
Unicef 15, 16
United Nations Environment
 Programme 29, 30
United Nations Population Fund 9, 17
United States
 bicycles 70
 catalytic converters 61

United States (*continued*)
 cataracts 31
 chlorofluorocarbons policy 32
 coastal bathing policy 102
 cycling 71
 deaths from asthma 56
 emissions policy 24
 grain harvest 9-10
 hearing damage 74
 lead in air and blood 61
 skin cancer 29
 x ray examinations 114
urban growth 14

vapour retrieval systems 62
vehicles 2
 cars 66, 67, 71
 emissions 3, 4, 24, 47
  carcinogenic 57
  diesel and petrol 59
  reduction 61-2
 growth in numbers 62
viruses, in sea water 101

waste 4
 burning 40
 clinical 34-7
 and disease 39
 industrial 38-40
waste disposal 34-43
 alternatives 41-2
water
 assessment of quality 88
 bottled 5, 90
 contamination by waste 40
 health risks 89-92
 irrigation 11-2
 quality 85-94
 river 86
 sea bathing, standards 100-2
 tap 5, 85, 90, 93
 treatment 86-7
water industry 85, 87-9, 93
Wheeler, David 100
Windscale 110
Wolff, Simon 57

x rays 113-5

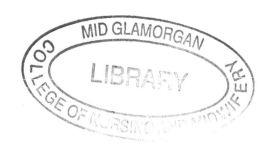